Anemia &
Heavy
Menstrual
Flow

❖ ❖ ❖

Anemia & Heavy Menstrual Flow

❖ ❖ ❖

Susan M. Lark, M.D.

Cover & Text Design: Brad Greene
Photographs: Ronald May
Illustrations: Shelly Reeves Smith
Printing & Binding: Arcata Graphics Company

𝒲estchester Publishing Company
342 State Street, Suite 6
Los Altos, CA 94022
415-941-5784

To my wonderful husband Jim and
my darling daughter Rebecca
To the health and well-being of all women

❖ ❖ ❖

Contents

Introduction

A Self-Help Approach to Anemia & Heavy Menstrual Flow

*T*his book on anemia and heavy menstrual flow is the third in a series of self-help books I am writing for women. For almost two decades I have worked with thousands of women who came to me as patients and as participants in my classes and seminars. They included teenagers, women in their reproductive years, pregnant women, menopausal women, and women well past their reproductive prime who were facing the health issues of old age. With all these women, I noted one trait in common: No matter what her age or health problems, regardless of her social or economic status, each had an intense desire for information on how to stay healthy and symptom-free.

In my medical practice, I have always combined information and education on self-care along with any medical treatments. After seeing so many of my patients become symptom-free over time, I am a firm believer in the power of self-care. Changing your lifestyle habits in beneficial ways gives your body the chance to heal itself. My goal as a physician is to help my patients become symptom-free, thereby reducing their need for medical care. I don't believe that an unfavorable medical diagnosis need be a lifetime sentence of poor health.

Any woman who is faced with the need to handle significant female-related problems finds an almost total lack of available information. Even on topics for which information is available, such as premenstrual syndrome and menopause, the books have primarily discussed only the symptoms of the problems and the standard medical treatments. Health-care providers and authors have supplied little in-depth information on what women can do on their own to maintain their health and well-being. As a physician specializing in women's health care and preventive medicine, I wrote this book to meet some of the needs that women have for more complete self-help information.

Anemia and heavy menstrual flow can affect women at many different times in their lives, causing significant symptoms and impairing the ability to handle day-to-day life in an optimal and competent way. Often these medical problems recur, and each time stronger and more powerful treatments may be needed to stop the process. Treatments include the use of medications, hormones, and surgical procedures, even to the point of a hysterectomy. Though these therapies are important and can even be life-saving in some cases, they may not be inevitable if the underlying causes of the health problems are looked at and treated in time. Each year approximately 800,000 women in this country undergo hysterectomies, many due to heavy menstrual bleeding. While some women clearly need this procedure because of life-threatening problems such as cancer, a large percentage could avoid surgery if the underlying causes of the problems were treated.

In many cases, the factors that put women at risk originate in their lifestyles. Our bodies have an amazing ability to heal if we treat them well. I have found through my years of practice that many women can prevent, or at least minimize, both anemia and heavy menstrual bleeding through proper self-help techniques that include specific dietary guidelines, as well as the right nutritional supplements, exercise programs, and stress-reduction techniques. Such steps can have dramatic beneficial effects for women suffering from anemia and heavy menstrual flow. Unfortunately, most of this exciting information lies buried in medical research journals and has not been made available to women who need it.

Self-help information is available in this book, and I hope you will find it as useful as my patients have. I practice these techniques, too. Preventive health care has provided tremendous benefits for me; I am healthier and more productive now than I was ten years ago. I plan to feel better and to be even healthier ten years from now. I continually expand my knowledge about self-help and constantly research new health-care techniques for anemia and heavy menstrual bleeding.

How To Use This Self-Help Book

This anemia and heavy menstrual flow self-help program provides very important information for all women suffering from these problems. I have written the program so that each woman reading this book can select from a wide variety of self-help treatment options. To this end, I have included many self-help techniques. A treatment plan based on only one method that purports to be the only treatment for anemia and heavy menstrual flow will probably work for only a small percentage of women. In my medical practice, I have found that results are much better if I completely individualize each patient's treatment program. By overlapping treatments from various disciplines, most women find combinations that work for them. You will be able to find a combination that works for you, too.

This program is set up so that you can develop your own treatment plan. All the methods you need are contained in this book, including information on diet and nutrition as well as beneficial vitamins, minerals, and herbs. Nutritional supplementation is a very important part of an optimal health program for any woman with anemia and heavy menstrual flow. I have also included suggestions for stress-reduction techniques, exercises for fitness and flexibility, acupressure massage, and yoga poses that are specifically helpful for symptoms arising from anemia and heavy menstrual bleeding.

First, read through the entire book to familiarize yourself with the material. The Workbook (Chapter 3) can help you evaluate your symptoms, and the Summary Treatment Chart for Anemia and Heavy Menstrual Flow (in Chapter 4) directs you to the treatments appropriate for your particular set of problems. These tools are quick and easy to use and will save you countless hours of work on your own. You can discover simply and easily what will work: Try all the therapies listed under your symptoms, and you will probably find that some make you feel better than others. On a regular basis, do those techniques that provide relief for your symptoms. Establish a regimen that works for you and use it every day.

This program is practical and easy to follow. It can be used by itself or in conjunction with a medical program. And best of all, it works. The feeling of wellness that can be yours with a self-help program will radiate and touch your whole life. You will have more time and energy to enjoy your work, family, and other pleasures. Most of my patients tell me that their lives have been positively transformed by following these beneficial self-help techniques.

Susan M. Lark, MD

Learning About
the Problem

❖   ❖   ❖

1

What Is Anemia?

*A*nemia is one of the most common health problems affecting women of all ages. It has been estimated that as many as 20 percent of all American women suffer from anemia. Anemia can be found in all age groups—from childhood to old age. It is not restricted in frequency to any one period of a woman's life. Anemia is characterized by a reduction in the number of red blood cells or a reduction in hemoglobin (the oxygen-carrying protein in red blood cells). Anemia reduces the amount of oxygen available to all cells of the body; then, carbon dioxide, a waste product, accumulates in the cells and cannot be removed by the lungs with normal respirations. As a result of the blood's lower oxygen-carrying capability, the cells for the body's normal chemical functioning have less available energy. Important processes, such as muscular activity and cell building and repair, slow down and become less efficient. Greater than 95 percent of the body's chemical reactions depend on optimal oxygen levels in cells and tissues. As a result, the symptoms of anemia can be very debilitating.

The Symptoms

The symptoms of anemia are numerous and affect many organ systems in the body. Often the symptoms seem vague and misleading to women and to their physicians. In fact, every symptom of anemia can be mistaken for other health conditions, including emotional problems and nervous tension. Because the lack of oxygen impairs the body's ability to carry out its numerous chemical reactions, many women with anemia feel extremely tired and fatigued. Because muscular activity is inhibited, they lack endurance and physical stamina. I have had many physically active patients who had to stop pursuing vigorous aerobic exercise programs when they developed anemia. These women simply lacked the physical energy to continue their active exercise regimens once the anemia became too severe.

When the brain cells lack oxygen, dizziness may result and mental faculties are less sharp. Women who are anemic tend to be pale with poor skin color and tone. They often appear "washed-out" and seem listless. They lack the glowing skin color that we tend to associate with good health and vitality. Women with anemia may also suffer from hair loss and brittle, ridged fingernails.

Digestive symptoms include loss of appetite, sore tongue, abdominal pain, heartburn, and diarrhea. In more severe cases, women can suffer from symptoms as varied as headaches, heart palpitations, tingling in the fingers and feet, loss of coordination, and a yellowing of the skin. As you can see, a woman can become quite ill from the physical and mental effects of anemia if her physician does not diagnose her condition properly.

Symptoms of Anemia

Fatigue
Dizziness
General weakness
Paleness
Loss of appetite
Brittle and ridged nails
Abdominal pain
Sore tongue

Yellowing of skin

Tingling in hands and feet

Loss of coordination

Diarrhea

How Red Blood Cells Are Formed

To understand anemia, you should first understand how normal red blood cells are produced. Then you can follow how the different types of anemia occur, particularly those due to nutritional deficiencies in which a lack of proper nutrients impairs the normal production of red blood cells.

Before birth, as we grow and mature in the uterus, our bodies have no specific centers for red cell production. Red cells are formed in many places: the yolk sac, spleen, liver, thymus gland, lymph nodes, and bone marrow. After birth and as we grow toward adulthood, the production of red cells shifts predominantly to the red bone marrow of certain bones, including the pelvis, vertebrae, ribs, sternum or chest bone, skull, and the humerus and femur (the bones of arms and legs).

The formation of new, immature red cells takes place in the bone marrow. The immature red cells go through several transformations before gaining the ability to produce hemoglobin, the oxygen-carrying protein found in red blood cells. After several more transformations in the bone marrow, the red blood cells mature to cells called reticulocytes. Reticulocytes contain about one-third of their weight in hemoglobin. At maturity, red blood cells lose their nuclei, or core; this transformation makes the cells more fluid and flexible. With this increased flexibility, the reticulocytes can leave the bone marrow and enter the bloodstream by squeezing through the walls of the small blood vessels or capillaries.

The mature red blood cell looks like a concave disk on both sides and has a very simple structure with no core or nucleus. It also lacks the ability to reproduce or carry on extensive chemical activities. The red blood cell has an outer cell membrane composed of protein that encloses the cell body (or cytoplasm) and the hemoglobin. The hemoglobin molecule consists of a protein called globin and a pigment called heme, which contains iron. Hemoglobin is a red-colored pigment that is responsible for the red color of the blood. As mentioned earlier, the hemoglobin allows the oxygen to attach to the red blood cells and be transported throughout the body. A healthy woman has about 4.7 million red blood cells per cubic millimeter of blood (a very small unit of volume), while a healthy man has about 5.4 million red blood cells per cubic millimeter of blood.

Since the life span of a red blood cell is only 120 days, the body constantly breaks down old red blood cells and forms new ones. In fact, the body produces an astonishing 2 million new red blood cells per second. The old red blood cells are destroyed in the liver and spleen, and these substances are either reused or eliminated from the body. If this process breaks down at any point, then anemia, or lack of red blood cells, can occur.

How Anemia Is Diagnosed

Health-care providers can diagnose anemia simply by removing a small sample of blood from the body and looking at the number and characteristics of the red blood cells. This is one of the most common medical tests done on patients in the United States. When evaluating the blood sample for anemia, the total number of red blood cells are counted. The percentage of blood that is made up of red blood cells, or the hematocrit, is also estimated by determining the ratio of red blood cells to the whole blood. In healthy women the hematocrit averages 38 to 47 percent; it is lower in women with anemia. In this blood test, the hemoglobin level, or amount of pigment in the blood, is commonly estimated also. For healthy women, the normal range is 12.0 to 15.0 grams per deciliter. Hemoglobin level, red blood cells, and hematocrit are all reduced in women with anemia.

Causes of Anemia

The most common cause of anemia is iron deficiency. When women are iron-deficient, their red blood cells do not mature properly and remain small and pale-colored. It has been estimated that as many as one-third to one-half of young American women have low or depleted iron stores. The main reason for these low reserves is that women simply don't eat enough iron-rich foods. Many women diet excessively, so their total caloric intake does not contain sufficient foods to sustain an adequate iron reserve. For some women, dairy products such as yogurt, cheese, and cottage cheese constitute their main source of protein. Dairy products are very low in iron content. Women who eat a lot of "junk foods" such as candy bars, chocolate, french fries, and other high-fat, high-sugar foods are also stacking their dietary intake toward inadequate amounts of iron. Women athletes also have an increased need for iron during training because of the metabolic demands of heavy exercise.

Children, adolescents, and women during their reproductive years require adequate iron. This iron is needed to support growth and development in children and teenage girls and to replace the iron lost in the monthly menstrual period during a woman's reproductive years. During an average menstrual period, it is estimated that a woman loses approximately 18 mg of iron through the loss of red blood cells. This equals a daily average iron loss of 0.6 mg over a month's time. As a result, women during their reproductive years need twice as much iron intake as men. This need persists until menopause, when the monthly blood loss finally ceases. Elderly women are still susceptible to developing anemia because they tend to eat less and have a nutrient-poor diet, which may be due to living alone or having a limited income.

Pregnancy and the postpartum period are also vulnerable times for women. During pregnancy, the volume of the mother's blood increases and the growing fetus has its own needs for iron. To meet these demands, pregnant women must increase their iron intake through iron supplementation as well as proper dietary habits. Nursing mothers need iron to build up the reserves that were depleted during pregnancy. Also, iron is lost through the breast milk because this important mineral is used to fortify the newborn infant and must be replaced by the lactating mother.

The official recommendations for iron intake at all phases of a woman's life are as follows:

Teenagers through reproductive years	15 mg per day
Pregnant women	30 mg per day
Nursing mothers	15 mg per day
Postmenopausal women	10 mg per day

Besides consuming an adequate amount of iron in your diet, you must also be able to absorb the iron properly. Even if you have an iron-rich diet, the lack of vitamin A or of B vitamins such as thiamine (B_1), riboflavin (B_2), niacin (B_3), and pantothenic acid (B_5) can result in an under- or nonabsorption of iron. Iron absorption is also decreased by chronic diarrhea, laxative abuse, and malabsorption diseases such as celiac disease and sprue. Vitamin C can be very helpful in facilitating iron absorption. At least 75 mg must be provided daily in the diet, either through a combination of fruits and vegetables or the use of a supplement. However, you should avoid calcium supplements and calcium carbonate-based antacids when you ingest iron supplements or iron-rich foods, because calcium inhibits iron absorption.

Another common reason for the development of iron deficiency anemia is excessive blood loss, such as that experienced by women who suffer from menorrhagia (heavy or prolonged menstrual bleeding). Menorrhagia is commonly seen in women with problems such as hormonal imbalances, fibroid tumors, and uterine cancer. Women who use intrauterine devices for contraception are also at higher risk of blood loss. In fact, it is estimated that 10 percent of women using IUDs have significant loss of blood, and therefore iron. The excessive use of anti-inflammatory medications such as aspirin or ibuprofen can cause blood loss through the digestive tract. This occurs because anti-inflammatory medication causes irritation of the stomach lining.

Iron is not the only mineral needed for healthy red blood cell production. Two other minerals, copper and zinc, also play important roles. Copper assists in the formation of hemoglobin and red blood cells by increasing iron absorption. Zinc deficiency has been found in people suffering from sickle-cell anemia. Clinical studies have shown that zinc supplementation helped decrease the number of sickled cells.

Pernicious anemia is another form of anemia caused by nutritional deficiencies, in this case, vitamin B_{12}. This deficiency can often be traced to the inability of the stomach to secrete the "intrinsic factor," a substance necessary for the absorption of vitamin B_{12}. The lack of the intrinsic factor is an inherited trait and results in a severe form of anemia in which the red blood cells do not grow and mature properly. The symptoms of vitamin B_{12} deficiency can be slow to appear once the body's supply of this nutrient diminishes, usually taking as long as four to six years once B_{12} stores are depleted. As a result of B_{12} deficiency, the body produces fewer red blood cells, and the red blood cells themselves are large and abnormally shaped. Vegetarians are also more prone to develop B_{12} deficiency, because this nutrient is found primarily in animal protein, such as liver. Persons who have this deficiency must receive B_{12} injections in order to avoid the serious symptoms that can result. Vitamin B_{12} deficiency can cause nervous system damage, mental disturbances, digestive symptoms, and slight yellowing of the skin.

Folic acid, another member of the vitamin B complex, is also needed for the production of healthy red blood cells. Folic acid is an essential factor in the formation of heme, the iron-containing pigment found in hemoglobin. As you recall, hemoglobin is the protein that carries oxygen in the red blood cells. Along with vitamin B_{12}, it plays an important role in the breakdown and utilization of proteins. Like vitamin B_{12}, a deficiency in folic acid hinders normal red blood cell production and creates large, abnormally shaped cells. Folic acid is also essential for healthy brain and nervous system function. Folic acid deficiencies are common in women, especially teenagers and elderly women, because of poor nutritional habits. Folic acid is found primarily in leafy green vegetables and liver, which do not figure significantly in many women's diets. Also, women who use birth control pills for contraception or to regulate their cycles are at higher risk of developing folic acid deficiency.

Pyridoxine, or vitamin B_6, is also necessary for normal red blood cell production. According to medical studies, anemia that fails to respond to iron may be corrected with daily supplementation of vitamin B_6. Other research suggests that patients with sickle-cell anemia have abnormally low levels of vitamin B_6 in their red blood cells, levels that may be raised by supplementation.

Though iron, vitamin B_{12}, folic acid, vitamin B_6, and many other nutrients are necessary for red blood cell production, vitamin E is important for red blood cell survival. Medical research done on subjects deficient in vitamin E has shown that this nutrient helps to prolong the life span of red blood cells. Vitamin E also seems to help extend the life of the red blood cells in patients with cystic fibrosis and other types of pancreatic disease.

Women Are at Risk of Anemia Throughout Their Lives

Teenagers

Menstruating Women

Pregnant Women

Nursing Mothers

Contraceptive Users: Intra-
     uterine Devices, Birth Control Pills

Athletic Women in Training

Elderly Women

Anemia is a problem that can complicate preexisting health-care conditions. For example, anemia often accompanies thyroid disease, rheumatoid arthritis, and chronic kidney disease, as well as infections that tend to recur and become chronic. Anemia contributes to the fatigue and lack of energy that affect people suffering from these health problems.

Some anemias are genetically linked and are more prevalent in certain ethnic groups. Sickle-cell anemia is found in people of African descent and can cause severe symptoms, including episodes of fever and pain in the arms, legs, and abdomen. These symptoms can start in early childhood and are due to a decrease in the fluidity of the whole blood, which causes a blood flow obstruction in the small blood vessels. Another type of genetically linked anemia is thalassemia, which is found primarily in people of Southeast Asian or Mediterranean heritage. In severe cases, thalassemia causes an enlarged liver and spleen, as well as a very low red blood cell count. Infant mortality among those severely affected is quite high.

Anemia can also be caused by drugs that destroy or interfere with the utilization of the nutrients necessary for the health and maturation of the red blood cells. These drugs include oral contraceptives, alcohol, and anticonvulsive agents such as Dilantin. Exposure to radiation or to toxic chemicals, such as certain insecticides, may also damage the bone marrow, resulting in anemia.

Causes of Anemia

Nutritional Deficiencies

Minerals:

    Iron, copper, zinc

Vitamins:

    A; B complex, especially
    folic acid, B_{12}, B_6; C; and E

Blood Loss

Excessive menstrual bleeding

Use of anti-inflammatory drugs

Intrauterine devices

Disease-Related Anemia

Thyroid disease

Rheumatoid arthritis

Kidney disease

Chronic infections

Malabsorption syndrome

Other chronic diseases

Environmental Toxicity

Toxic chemical exposure

Radiation poisoning

Drug intake

2

What Is Heavy Menstrual Flow?

*O*ne of the most common reasons for anemia, other than nutritional deficiencies, is heavy menstrual bleeding. This condition is usually called "menorrhagia" by your physician and refers to blood loss that occurs either in a rapid, heavy flow or in a more moderate flow over an unusually long period of time. Blood loss is not always limited to the duration of the menstrual cycle; some women spot between periods. Spotting also occasionally happens at midcycle as an accompaniment to "mittelschmerz," or the slight pain that occurs at ovulation.

Heavy, profuse menstrual bleeding can be an uncomfortable experience. Some women need to use double pads or a pad and a tampon and must change them frequently, as often as every hour or two in severe cases. Many times, even frequent changes of pads and tampons do not soak up all the blood loss. Excessive menstrual flow can stain underwear and clothing, often at the most inopportune times, which can obviously be unpleasant and embarrassing. Profuse menstrual flow can also be accompanied by large blood clots, which can be painful to pass and may leave a woman feeling weak, fatigued, and literally drained of energy for a day or two each month. If this process is allowed to go untreated, the excessive blood loss over time can lead to anemia.

The Normal Menstrual Cycle

Let us look at the normal menstrual cycle and see how it functions. This information will make it much easier for you to understand the changes that can occur to disrupt this normal pattern and cause excessive menstrual bleeding.

First, it is important to understand why menstruation occurs. Menstruation refers to the shedding of the uterine lining, or endometrium. Each month the uterus prepares a thick, blood-rich cushion to nourish and house a fertilized egg. If conception occurs, the endometrium becomes the placenta. If pregnancy doesn't occur, the egg doesn't implant in the uterus and the body doesn't need the extra buildup of uterine lining. The uterus cleanses itself by releasing the extra blood and tissue so that the buildup can recur the following month.

The mechanism that regulates the buildup and shedding of the uterine lining is controlled by fluctuations in hormonal levels. Fluctuations are based on a feedback system in which the pituitary gland secretes a chemical, or hormone. The hormone enters the bloodstream where it circulates to a target gland—an ovary. The hormone acts as a messenger, instructing the target gland to make its own hormone. In other cases, the hormone can trigger chemical reactions in other parts of the body.

Let's look at the way this feedback system operates in the menstrual cycle. Three glands are directly involved in turning menstruation on and off: the hypothalamus, the pituitary, and the ovaries. Other glands, such as the adrenals and thyroid, are also necessary for healthy menstrual function.

The initial trigger for the menstrual cycle comes from hormones produced in the hypothalamus, a walnut-sized collection of highly specialized brain cells located above the pituitary. The hypothalamus regulates many basic bodily functions besides the production of female sex hormones, including temperature control, sleep patterns, thirst, and hunger. The hypothalamus is very sensitive to stresses such as emotional problems and infections. Severe stresses can affect the ability of the hypothalamus to pass signals to the pituitary and from there to the other endocrine glands. This can cause imbalances in the menstrual cycle.

The pituitary, located at the base of the brain, stimulates all the glands of the body and provides the next mechanism in regulating the menstrual cycle. To communicate with the pituitary, the hypothalamus releases messengers into the bloodstream called FSH-RF (follicle-stimulating hormone–releasing factor) and LH-RF (luteinizing hormone–releasing factor). When these messages from the hypothalamus are received, the pituitary begins to produce its own hormones. It triggers the menstrual cycle and ovulation by secreting FSH (follicle-stimulating hormone) and LH (luteinizing hormone). It also triggers adrenal function through the production of ACTH (adrenocorticotrophic hormone) and thyroid function through TSH (thyroid-stimulating hormone).

Once FSH and LH are released into the bloodstream, their destinations are the ovaries, the female reproductive organ. The ovaries are two small, almond-shaped glands located in a woman's pelvis. The ovaries hold all the eggs a woman will ever have, in an inactive form called follicles. At birth, each female has about 1 million follicles. By puberty, the number of eggs has been reduced to 300,000 to 400,000. The eggs decrease in number throughout a woman's life, until menopause, at which time the follicles have atrophied and lost their ability to produce estrogen. Without sufficient estrogen, menstruation ceases.

Each month, FSH and LH from the pituitary cause the follicles to ripen and release an egg for possible fertilization. (Usually only one ovary is stimulated in a cycle.) In doing so, the follicles begin to produce the hormones estrogen and progesterone. Estrogen reaches its peak during the first half of the cycle, while progesterone output occurs after midcycle when ovulation has occurred. Ovulation refers to the production of a mature egg cell, which travels down the fallopian tube to the uterus. Fertilization normally occurs in the fallopian tube. Besides preparing the egg for fertilization, estrogen and progesterone stimulate the lining of the uterus.

During the first two weeks following menstruation, estrogen causes the uterine lining to gradually rebuild itself. The glands of the endometrium begin to grow long and the lining thickens through an increase in the number of blood vessels as well as the production of a mesh of fibers that interconnect throughout the lining. By midcycle, the lining of the uterus has increased three times in thickness and has a greatly increased blood supply.

After midcycle, usually around day 14, ovulation occurs and the egg is picked up by a fallopian tube for the journey to the uterus. The follicle that produced the egg for that month (or Graafian follicle) is further stimulated after midcycle by LH and changes into the yellow body, or *corpus luteum*. The *corpus luteum* secretes progesterone—the second ovarian hormone of the menstrual cycle—which causes a coiling of the blood vessels of the uterine lining. The uterine lining becomes swollen and tortuous and secretes a thick mucous.

If the egg is fertilized, it will implant on the uterine wall and the *corpus luteum* will continue to secrete progesterone. If no fertilization occurs, the *corpus luteum* begins to deteriorate and the progesterone levels decrease. The lining of the uterus starts to break down and menstruation begins.

What Causes Heavy Menstrual Bleeding?

A number of conditions can cause excessive bleeding. It occurs frequently at either end of the reproductive cycle—in puberty and during perimenopause (the time of transition into menopause). During adolescence, a woman's estrogen levels are gradually increasing. While her menstrual cycle is in the process of establishing itself on a mature adult basis, ovulation is often infrequent or sporadic. As a result, an adolescent may have periods that are heavier, longer, or closer together than those of adult women. Menstrual cycles that occur without ovulation are called anovulatory cycles. After a few years of menstruation, this pattern of heavy menstrual bleeding tends to self-correct as ovulation begins to occur on a regular basis.

At the other end of the spectrum, as women approach menopause, their follicles gradually atrophy and diminish in number. This transition period can last as long as four to five years. As their follicles lose the ability to produce estrogen and progesterone, perimenopausal women begin to ovulate less frequently. For many women, the transitions into menopause can be uncomfortable and difficult experiences. As the hormonal output becomes unstable during a woman's mid to late forties, irregular heavy bleeding may occur. The menstrual cycle often shortens, with periods coming closer together. Bleeding may become heavier and last longer. A one-week to ten-day menstrual period is fairly common. Some patients tell me that their cycles are unpredictable, sometimes coming twice a month, and in some extreme cases lasting as long as 60 or more days. This blood loss can be dangerous because it can lead to anemia if not treated. As with most menstrual problems that women encounter while entering adolescence, unpredictable cycles eventually correct themselves. When menopause approaches, the periods occur at longer intervals and the flow becomes light and scanty until menstruation finally ceases.

During a phase of heavy menstrual bleeding, women are likely to need medical care. Often the bleeding can be stopped by a synthetic progesterone-like hormone called a progestin. Provera is the type used most often in the United States. Provera can be administered by mouth for one or two weeks and usually stops the bleeding. It acts in much the same way as natural progesterone, limiting the amount of bleeding from the uterine lining during the second half of the menstrual cycle.

For some women, the use of progestins is not sufficient, and an operation called a dilatation and curettage (D&C) must be done. The D&C effectively stops the bleeding by removing the lining of the uterus through a scraping or suction technique while the patient is under anesthesia. The D&C is useful in ruling out other, potentially more serious, causes of bleeding. After the D&C, cells of the uterine lining can be analyzed for abnormalities such as uterine polyps or cancer.

If the bleeding is found to be due only to the hormonal instability that occurs prior to menopause, the symptoms may recur throughout the transition into menopause. Women are most likely to have a hysterectomy performed during this time. Over 800,000 hysterectomies are done each year in the United States. Interestingly enough, only 10 to 12 percent are done for life-threatening reasons, such as cancer. During the 18 years of my practice, I have found that many cases of heavy menstrual bleeding can be treated in a conservative, nonsurgical fashion by employing supportive therapy such as nutrition and stress management and, as necessary, hormonal therapy. If a woman with heavy menstrual bleeding due to hormonal instability can get through the transition period and avoid a hysterectomy, the problem will often self-correct with menopause, and the woman will have avoided major surgery. Of course, this is not always possible, and there are cases of serious profuse bleeding in which a hysterectomy may be the only sensible and correct solution.

You should be aware that menstrual bleeding is affected by many environmental factors. For example, cigarette smoking and excessive alcohol intake can worsen menstrual bleeding. Alcohol, if used in excess, is toxic to the liver. The liver is responsible for the breakdown of the estrogen so that it can be excreted from the body. If the liver is not functioning properly, the circulating levels of estrogen may be too high and thus worsen the bleeding problem.

Stress of all kinds can worsen menstrual bleeding. The menstrual cycle is ultimately dependent on the smooth functioning of the endocrine glands. As mentioned earlier, the normal functioning of the hypothalamus in the brain is strongly affected by major stresses of any kind. Traumas such as divorce, death of a loved one, job changes, moving to a new home, or even taking a major trip can impact the menstrual cycle of a susceptible woman. Helpful techniques to deal with stress are included in the self-help section of this book.

Regular menstrual cycles depend not only on emotional health but also on good nutritional habits. Women who are grossly overweight produce higher levels of estrogen and are at greater risk of anovulatory cycles and heavy menstrual bleeding. For these women, a low-fat, low-sugar diet is mandatory. An optimal diet will contain plenty of high-nutrient foods, such as whole grains, beans, peas, fresh fruits and vegetables, raw seeds and nuts, and fish (for women who eat meat as a main form of protein). Women who eat a nutrient-poor diet are also at high risk of heavy menstrual bleeding because they lack the nutrients to regulate normal blood flow. Medical studies have shown that deficiencies of vitamin A, vitamin C, iron, and bioflavonoids can worsen or even cause heavy, irregular menstrual bleeding. These nutrients should be included in both the diets and supplement programs of women with heavy bleeding. The self-help section of this book provides detailed information on foods, vitamins, minerals, and herbs that help to control heavy menstrual flow.

While many cases of heavy menstrual flow are due to hormonal imbalances, other medical problems can also cause bleeding. One of the most common is fibroid tumors. Fibroids, also called myomas, are benign growths of muscle and connective tissue, usually found in the wall of the uterus. They are a common condition affecting 20 to 50 percent of all women. For many women, fibroids do not create a problem because the tumors tend to be small and don't cause any symptoms. However, for some women in their thirties and forties, fibroids can become a real problem. In these women, the fibroids either grow to be so large or become so numerous that they put pressure on the bowel or bladder wall, causing discomfort, frequent urination, and changes in bowel habits. At times, the fibroids grow to be so large that a woman feels them in her uterus through the abdominal wall, and she can appear to be four to five months pregnant. Sometimes fibroids outgrow their blood supply, causing much discomfort. Fibroids can also cause heavy menstrual bleeding, which can lead to anemia.

Fibroids are one of the most common causes of hysterectomies in American women. Like the heavy menstrual bleeding seen in perimenopausal women, fibroids are stimulated by unopposed high levels of estrogen. For this reason, women with fibroids should avoid birth control pills, estrogen replacement therapy after menopause, alcohol, high-fat diets, and excessive life stresses, since these factors can stimulate high levels of estrogen. Vitamin E, vitamin B complex, and herbs that have low levels of progesterone or help optimize liver function may be helpful in treating fibroids. Information about diet and supplements that are helpful for fibroids can be found in the self-help section of this book.

Because fibroids are stimulated by estrogen, they tend to shrink in size after menopause. If a woman can avoid having a hysterectomy during the transition period, she may have no further problems once menstruation ends. For women whose symptoms require a surgical treatment for their fibroids, several options are available. A young woman who wishes to have children at a later date may elect to have a myomectomy, a procedure that removes only the fibroids. This may relieve the pain and bleeding, but further surgery may be needed later if the fibroids continue to grow. Women who are past their childbearing years and have uncomfortable bowel or bladder symptoms or severe bleeding may require a hysterectomy. However, unless the fibroids actually cause symptoms or show signs of malignancy (which is very rare), they do not need to be removed. In my opinion, many gynecologists recommend hysterectomies that are unnecessary.

Other abnormal uterine growths are stimulated by excessive levels of estrogen and can cause profuse bleeding as the initial symptom. Overgrowth of the uterine lining (endometrial hyperplasia) and uterine (endometrial) cancer tend to be seen in older women or those who are in transition into menopause. Risk factors associated with cancerous or precancerous growths of the uterus include obesity, hypertension, diabetes mellitus, childlessness, and a history of breast cancer. Using unopposed estrogen without progesterone for postmenopausal hormonal replacement therapy increases a woman's risk of developing uterine cancer fivefold. Dietary and stress factors also increase the risk of excessive estrogen levels. Cancer of the uterus and precancerous lesions are linked to excessive bleeding before, during, or after menstruation, as well as postmenopausal bleeding and spotting. Bleeding in a postmenopausal woman should be evaluated carefully to find the possible cause.

Evaluating
Your Symptoms

❖   ❖   ❖

3

The Anemia &
Heavy Menstrual Flow
Workbook

*T*his workbook section will help you evaluate your symptoms as well as the factors that contribute to your risk of developing anemia and heavy menstrual bleeding. It is important to be aware of your risk factors since these problems can recur throughout your reproductive years and, in the case of anemia, well into your postmenopausal years. Luckily, you can eliminate many risk factors by modifying your lifestyle habits.

If you take the time to fill out the evaluation sheets, you'll find it easier to recognize your weak areas; then you can put together your own treatment program from the following chapters for the best relief and prevention of anemia and heavy menstrual bleeding.

First, fill out the checklist to evaluate your symptoms. Then, carefully assess your responses for the risk factors for anemia and heavy menstrual bleeding. Finally, fill out the lifestyle habit evaluations related to eating and exercise. These will help you assess specific areas of your life to see which of your habit patterns are contributing to your symptoms. This evaluation will also show you if you are at risk for anemia or heavy menstrual bleeding. Working with the preventive health-care techniques in the rest of the book can help improve your health and lessen your risks.

When you have completed the evaluations, you will be ready to go on to the next chapter and begin your treatment program.

Symptoms of Anemia & Heavy Menstrual Flow

The most common symptoms of anemia are listed below. The first four symptoms may occur in women with heavy menstrual bleeding. Check those that pertain to you. Some women have very few symptoms, while others have symptoms severe enough to affect their ability to function normally. The worse your symptoms, the more important it is that you follow the self-help guidelines in this book.

	Yes	No
Fatigue	___	___
Dizziness	___	___
General weakness	___	___
Paleness	___	___
Profuse or extended menstrual bleeding	___	___
Loss of appetite	___	___
Brittle nails	___	___
Abdominal pain	___	___
Sore tongue	___	___
Yellowing of skin	___	___
Tingling in hands and feet	___	___
Loss of coordination	___	___
Diarrhea	___	___

Risk Factors for Anemia

You may have a higher likelihood of developing anemia if any of the following risk factors are positive. Women are especially vulnerable to developing anemia at certain times in their lives, such as adolescence, pregnancy, and premenopause. During these phases of your life, careful attention to prevention may be helpful. Risk factors linked to lifestyle issues, such as poor diet and nutrient intake, can be easily modified; see the nutritional section of this book.

	Yes	No
Poor nutritional habits (high level of junk-food intake)	___	___
Iron-poor diet	___	___
Dietary lack of folic acid, vitamin B_{12}, other B complex vitamins, vitamins A, C, and E, copper, and zinc from either food or supplements *(If you are not sure which foods contain these nutrients, check the dietary chapter in this book.)*	___	___
High dairy-product diet	___	___
High wheat diet	___	___
Malabsorption syndrome, celiac disease, or sprue	___	___
Teenager	___	___
Heavy menstruation	___	___
Pregnancy	___	___
Peptic ulcer	___	___
Chronic use of laxatives	___	___
Chronic diarrhea	___	___
Vegetarian without dietary or supplemental source of vitamin B_{12}	___	___
Member of certain ethnic group (i.e., African American, Mediterranean, or Chinese)	___	___

Risk Factors for Heavy Menstrual Bleeding

You are at higher risk of heavy menstrual bleeding if you have any of the risk factors listed below. Be sure to follow the nutritional and other self-help techniques for uterine health. Get regular Pap smears. See your doctor if you have any abnormal vaginal bleeding after menopause because this bleeding can be a sign of uterine cancer.

	Yes	No
Lack of ovulation	____	____
Perimenopausal woman (in transition into menopause)	____	____
Fibroid tumors	____	____
Thyroid disease	____	____
Blood coagulation problem	____	____
Uterine polyps	____	____
Menopausal woman using estrogen replacement therapy without progesterone	____	____
Obesity	____	____
Early menstruation	____	____
Childlessness	____	____
High blood pressure	____	____
Lack of iodine	____	____
Lack of iron	____	____
Lack of vitamin A	____	____
Lack of vitamin C	____	____
Lack of bioflavonoids	____	____

Lifestyle Habits for Anemia & Heavy Menstrual Flow

Eating Habits

Check the number of times you eat the following foods:

Food	Never	Once a month	Once a week	Twice a week +
Coffee				
Black tea				
Soft drinks				
Cow's milk				
Cow's cheese				
Butter				
Yogurt				
Chocolate				

Food	Never	Once a month	Once a week	Twice a week +
Sugar				
Alcohol				
Pork				
Lamb				
White bread				
White noodles				
White flour pastries				
Added salt				
Bouillon				
Bottled salad dressing				
Catsup				
Hot dogs				
Bologna				
Salami				

Foods in shaded area are "high-stress" foods.

Avocado				
Beans				
Beets				
Broccoli				
Brussels sprouts				
Cabbage				
Carrots				
Celery				
Collard greens				
Cucumbers				
Eggplant				
Garlic				
Horseradish				
Kale				
Lettuce				
Mustard greens				
Okra				

Food	Never	Once a month	Once a week	Twice a week +
Onions				
Parsnips				
Peas				
Potatoes				
Radishes				
Rutabagas				
Spinach				
Squash				
Tomatoes				
Turnips				
Turnip greens				
Yams				
Almonds				
Filberts				
Peanuts				
Pecans				
Walnuts				
Barley				
Brown rice				
Buckwheat				
Corn				
Millet				
Oatmeal				
Pumpkin seeds				
Rye				
Sesame seeds				
Sunflower seeds				
Apples				
Apricots				
Bananas				
Berries				
Grapefruit				
Grapes				

Food	Never	Once a month	Once a week	Twice a week +
Melons				
Peaches				
Oranges				
Papayas				
Pears				
Pineapples				
Seasonal fruits				
Flax oil				
Olive oil				
Sesame oil				
Safflower oil				
Eggs				
Liver				
Fish				
Poultry				
Wild game (venison)				

Key to Eating Habits

Anemia and heavy menstrual bleeding tendencies are greatly affected by the quality of your nutritional habits: The production of healthy red blood cells and the ability to regulate menstrual flow depend on an abundance of nutrients such as iron, vitamin B_{12}, folic acid, vitamin B_6, vitamin E, bioflavonoids, and vitamin C, as well as other essential nutrients.

All foods on the preceding list from avocados to wild game are high-nutrient, low-stress foods. Many contain one or more of the essential nutrients needed to relieve and prevent anemia and heavy menstrual bleeding.

All foods in the shaded area are high-stress foods that can worsen your anemia and menstrual bleeding problems. If you eat large numbers of these foods, or if you eat any of these foods frequently, your nutritional habits may be contributing significantly to your symptoms, and you can probably benefit greatly from the dietary guidelines in the nutritional chapters. In fact, hard-to-digest foods such as wheat and dairy products may even make your anemia worse. This is because they can have a detrimental effect on absorption and assimilation of essential nutrients, such as iron, that are needed for the production of healthy red blood cells.

Exercise Habits

Check the number of times you do each of the following activities:

Activity	Never	Once a month	Once a week	Twice a week +
Walking				
Swimming				
Bicycling				
Stretching				
Yoga				
Golf				
Weight lifting (low stress)				
T'ai chi				
Ballroom dancing				

Key to Exercise Habits

Many women with anemia and heavy menstrual bleeding tend to have major problems with fatigue as well as lack of physical endurance and stamina. Even women who have been used to an active and vigorous exercise regimen may feel that any physical activity at all is just too difficult and may decide to stop exercising completely. This can have negative physiological effects on the body and increase the symptoms. While vigorous exercise may indeed exhaust a woman suffering from anemia, gentle and moderate exercise can provide the benefits of oxygenation and improved blood circulation. Select one or two of the less strenuous exercises given in the checklist and do them two to three times per week. Chapters 9 and 10 describe gentle exercise routines that you may find pleasant and easy to do.

Areas of Tension

Check the places where tension most commonly localizes in your body:

Location	Never	Seldom	Often	Always
Shoulders				
Neck and throat				
Grinding teeth				
Lower back				
Headache				
Eyestrain				
Arms				
Stomach muscles				

Key to Areas of Tension

This evaluation should help you become aware of how anemia and heavy menstrual flow can affect muscle tension in your body. Each woman has her own particular area where she localizes muscle tension. Anemia and heavy menstrual bleeding make less oxygen available to all the tissues of the body. There is a resultant accumulation of carbon dioxide and lactic acid. These waste products cause muscle contraction, as well as an increase in your level of fatigue and a decrease in your sense of vitality.

Try to remain aware of the areas in your body where you store tension. When you feel tension building up in them, do the stretches and stress-reduction exercises described in this book. They will help to reduce the tension significantly.

Stress Symptoms

Check the degree to which you are affected by the following symptoms:

	Never	Mildly	Moderately	Severely
Dizziness				
Decreased mental acuity				
Feeling constantly stressed				
Tension				
Mood swings				
Fatigue				
Depression				
Hopelessness				
Low self-esteem				

Key to Stress Symptoms

Women with both anemia and heavy menstrual bleeding may notice changes in their emotional state because of the fatigue and low energy that accompany these conditions. As a result of fatigue, feelings of hopelessness and depression may occur. If you have any of these symptoms, look at the many self-help treatment options described in this book. Try several of them and see which ones make you feel the best.

Finding
the Solution

❖ ❖ ❖

4

Self-Help Program—
A Summary Treatment
Chart

 $\mathcal{N}$ ow that you have read about the symptoms and causes of anemia and heavy menstrual bleeding, you are ready to put together your own self-help treatment program. I have included in this part of the book many treatment methods that I have found to be helpful with my patients. These treatment options include dietary and nutritional supplement programs as well as programs for stress management, exercise, acupressure, and yoga. Each of the following chapters presents specific information and techniques to help relieve and prevent anemia and heavy menstrual bleeding.

The program is set up so that you can individualize a treatment plan for yourself. This chapter contains a summary chart that will help you put your own program together. The chart lists all the treatments in this book that you can use for anemia and heavy menstrual bleeding.

There are two ways that you might use the summary chart. First, you can identify your problem in the chart and turn directly to the treatments for the problem. I recommend that when beginning a program, you try all the therapies listed for your problem. You will probably find that some techniques make you feel better than others. Establish the regimen that works for you and practice it on a regular basis. Alternatively, you can read straight through the rest of the book to get a general overview of the various treatment techniques. Find the treatments that you are interested in trying; then use the treatment chart for an overview and quick spot work.

Either way of working with the book can bring you tremendous benefits. The most important thing is to follow your program on a regular basis. This will enable you to see improvement in your health and vitality very quickly—many women begin to feel better within a month or two.

Summary Treatment Chart for
Anemia and Heavy Menstrual Bleeding

	Anemia	Heavy Menstrual Bleeding
Medication	Thyroid medication, anti-infection agents, medications for specific chronic disease problems	Progestins
Vitamins and Minerals	Anemia formula, with emphasis on iron, folic acid, vitamin B_{12}, vitamin B_6, vitamin C, and vitamin E	Heavy bleeding formula with emphasis on vitamin A, vitamin C, bioflavonoids, and iron
Herbs	Shepherd's purse, pau d'arco, yellow dock, golden seal, hawthorn berry, grape skins, cherry, bilberry, huckleberry, Oregon grape, licorice root	Shepherd's purse, golden seal, silymarin, curcumin, wild yam, hawthorn berry, grape skins, cherry, bilberry, huckleberry, Oregon grape
Nutrition	Anemia and heavy bleeding self-help diet	Anemia and heavy bleeding self-help diet
Stress Reduction	Stress reduction exercises 1, 2, 3, 4, 6	Stress reduction exercises 1, 3, 5, 7
Exercise	Exercises 1, 2, 3	Exercises 1, 2, 3
Yoga	Stretches 1, 2, 3, 4	Stretches 1, 2, 3, 4
Acupressure	Acupressure exercises 1, 2, 3, 4, 5	Acupressure exercises 1, 2, 3, 4, 5

5

Vitamins, Minerals, & Herbs

$\mathcal{T}$he use of vitamins, minerals, and herbs is extremely important for both the treatment and the prevention of anemia and heavy menstrual bleeding. In order to be symptom-free, you must have an optimal intake of the nutrients necessary for the growth and production of red blood cells and for the regulation of bleeding. I have found that my patients heal most effectively when they combine a nutrient-rich diet with the right mix of supplements. Though nothing can replace a healthful diet, most women have difficulty using diet alone to increase their nutrient intake to the levels needed for optimal healing. The use of supplements can help correct this deficiency so you can heal as rapidly and completely as possible.

As you read this chapter, you will learn about the beneficial effects that nutrition can have on fatigue, depression, low energy, poor digestion, and other symptoms of anemia and heavy menstrual bleeding. In fact, poor or inadequate nutrition may play a major role in causing these problems or contribute greatly to their onset. This chapter is divided into three sections. The first discusses the role of vitamins and minerals in the body, along with their major food sources. The next section tells which herbs are helpful for anemia and heavy menstrual bleeding and why they are effective. The third section gives specific recommendations on how to use these supplements, with one formula for anemia and another for heavy menstrual bleeding. Toward the end of the chapter I have included several charts listing major food sources of each essential nutrient. The importance of nutrition in regulating anemia and heavy menstrual bleeding is supported by numerous medical studies done at university centers and hospitals; a bibliography is included at the end of this chapter for those wanting more technical information.

Vitamins and Minerals for Anemia & Heavy Menstrual Bleeding

Vitamin A: Vitamin A is necessary for the normal growth and support of the eyes, skin, and mucous membranes and healthy immune function. Deficiency of vitamin A results in impaired immune function; rough, scaly skin; and night blindness. It is also needed for the healthy production of red blood cells. In an interesting study of middle-aged men on a diet deficient in vitamin A, it was found that the hemoglobin count started to decline even before a change in night vision or a measurable deficiency in the vitamin A levels was noted. Vitamin A also plays a significant role in the prevention of heavy menstrual bleeding. In a study of 71 women with excessive bleeding, the women were found to have significantly lower blood levels of vitamin A than the normal population. Almost 90 percent of the women studied returned to a normal bleeding pattern after two weeks of vitamin A treatment.

There are two types of vitamin A. Vitamin A from animal sources usually comes from fish liver and is oil soluble. This type of vitamin A can be toxic if taken in too large a dose (i.e., greater than 25,000 international units [I.U.] per day, if taken for more than a few months). In contrast, beta carotene, the precursor of vitamin A found in plants, is water soluble and is not toxic in large amounts. A single sweet potato or cup of carrot juice contains more than 20,000 I.U. of beta carotene.

Vitamin B Complex: The vitamin B complex consists of eleven factors that work together to perform many important biochemical functions in the body. These functions include stabilization of brain chemistry, glucose metabolism, and the inactivation of estrogen by the liver. Since heavy menstrual bleeding can be due to excess estrogen in the body, it is important that estrogen levels are properly regulated through breakdown and disposal by the liver. Vitamin B factors are essential for healthy liver functioning.

The B-complex vitamins are also necessary for the prevention and reversal of anemia. A deficiency of vitamin B_1 (thiamine), vitamin B_2 (riboflavin), vitamin B_5 (pantothenic acid), and vitamin B_6 (pyridoxine) may cause anemia, even in people who have no deficiencies in iron, folic acid, or vitamin B_{12}. The B-complex vitamins are commonly found in foods such as whole grains, beans and peas, and liver. These vitamins are water soluble. When a woman is under emotional stress, the B-complex vitamins are more easily lost from the body. This can worsen the fatigue and lack of vitality from which women with anemia and heavy menstrual bleeding already suffer.

Folic Acid: Folic acid is one of the B-complex vitamins and is an important nutrient for women. It helps prevent cervical dysplasia, a condition that can be a precursor to cancer of the cervix. It is also a necessary supplement for women who use birth control pills, since oral contraceptives interfere with folic acid absorption. Deficiency of folic acid in pregnant women has been linked to neural tube defects in their babies, such as spina bifida. Folic acid plays an important role in the production of red blood cells. A deficiency of folic acid leads to anemia that cannot be corrected by supplemental iron. With folic acid deficiency, red blood cells do not mature properly; they are large and irregularly shaped. Drugs that interfere with proper folic acid absorption include sulfa drugs and other antibiotics, phenobarbital, alcohol, and anticonvulsants used in the treatment of epilepsy. Women with folic acid deficiency anemia are prone to symptoms such as sore tongue, digestive disturbances, forgetfulness, and mental confusion. Good food sources of folic acid include oysters, salmon, whole grains, and green leafy vegetables.

Vitamin B_{12}: Vitamin B_{12} is a water-soluble vitamin that plays an important role in the production of red blood cells. Like folic acid deficiency, a B_{12} deficiency causes retardation in the growth and development of the red blood cells. B_{12}-deficient cells are immature and can develop only to a certain point. As with folic acid deficiency, these cells are large and abnormally shaped. Vitamin B_{12} is poorly absorbed from the gastrointestinal tract if the intrinsic factor, a necessary enzyme, is deficient. Since vitamin B_{12} is found primarily in meat, vegetarians may be at risk of developing a B_{12} deficiency. Symptoms of this deficiency develop slowly and may not become apparent for as long as five or six years after the body's supply of B_{12} has been restricted. A lack of B_{12} causes brain and nervous system damage. Symptoms include shooting pains, pins-and-needles or hot-and-cold sensations in the extremities, as well as numbness, stiffness, and difficulty in walking. This deficiency can also cause mental disturbances similar to psychosis, as well as memory defects and mental slowness. In order to treat B_{12} deficiency anemia (also known as pernicious anemia), the digestive tract must be bypassed and the B_{12} given as injections. When administered this way, B_{12} is an effective treatment for pernicious anemia.

Vitamin C: This important antistress vitamin is necessary for proper adrenal function as well as for immune function. Thus, large amounts of vitamin C are found in the adrenal glands. Vitamin C markedly increases iron absorption from the non-heme iron sources such as bran, peas, seeds, nuts, and leafy green vegetables. This can help to prevent iron deficiency anemia. Vitamin C has also been tested, along with bioflavonoids, as a treatment for heavy menstrual bleeding. One study showed a reduction in bleeding in 87 percent of the women participating. Vitamin C helps to strengthen capillaries and prevent capillary fragility, which can lead to excessive bleeding. Many fruits and vegetables are excellent sources of vitamin C.

Bioflavonoids: This is one of the most important nutrients for women at mid-life. Bioflavonoids have chemical activity similar to estrogen and can be used as an estrogen substitute. Clinical studies have shown that bioflavonoids help to control hot flashes and the psychological symptoms of menopause, including anxiety, irritability, and mood swings. Interestingly, bioflavonoids contain a very low potency of estrogen, much lower than that used as hormonal replacement therapy. As a result, no harmful side effects have been noted with bioflavonoid therapy.

Bioflavonoids have also shown dramatic results in their ability to reduce heavy menstrual bleeding through strengthening the capillary walls. They have been used in women with bleeding due to hormonal imbalance and have even been tested in women who have lost multiple pregnancies due to bleeding. They were used along with vitamin C in these studies. In nature, bioflavonoids can often be found with vitamin C in fruits and vegetables. For example, they are found in grape skins, cherries, blackberries, and blueberries. Bioflavonoids are also abundant in citrus fruits, especially in the pulp and the white rind.

Vitamin E: Vitamin E can act as an estrogen substitute. Like bioflavonoids, it has been studied as a treatment for hot flashes, the psychological symptoms of menopause, and even vaginal dryness in those women who either can't take or can't tolerate estrogen. In one study, vitamin E was found to help skew the estrogen-progesterone ratio in the body toward progesterone. This could be very helpful for those women who have heavy menstrual bleeding due to excess estrogen.

Vitamin E is also an important antioxidant. It protects the cells from the destructive effects of environmental pollutants that can react with the cell membrane. It has been found to increase red blood cell survival and, for this reason, is an important nutrient for the prevention of anemia. Vitamin E is found abundantly in wheat germ, nuts, seeds, and some fruits and vegetables.

Iron: Women who suffer from heavy menstrual bleeding tend to be iron deficient. In fact, some medical studies have found that inadequate iron intake may be a cause of excessive bleeding as well as an effect of the problem. Women who suffer from heavy menstrual bleeding should have their red blood count checked to see if supplemental iron is necessary, in addition to adopting a high-iron-content diet.

Heme iron, the iron from meat sources such as liver, is much better absorbed and assimilated than non-heme iron, the iron from vegetarian sources. To be absorbed properly, non-heme iron must be taken with at least 75 milligrams of vitamin C. For more information about food combinations that are high in both iron and vitamin C, see the following two chapters on dietary planning.

Iron deficiency is the main cause of anemia. Iron is an essential component of red blood cells, combining with protein and copper to make hemoglobin, the pigment of the red blood cells. Iron deficiency is common during all phases of a woman's life and is a frequent cause of fatigue and low-energy states. Good food sources of iron include liver, blackstrap molasses, beans and peas, seeds and nuts, and certain fruits and vegetables.

Copper: Copper aids in the formation of red blood cells. A deficiency of copper is associated with anemia, since copper is necessary for proper iron absorption. Copper is found in all body tissues and is present in many of the enzymes that break down and build up body tissues. The best food sources of copper include liver, whole grains, legumes, seafood, and green leafy vegetables.

Zinc: Zinc plays an important role in the body. It is a constituent of many enzymes involved both in metabolism and digestion. It is also needed for the proper growth and development of female reproductive organs and for the normal functioning of the male prostate gland. Good food sources of zinc include wheat germ, pumpkin seeds, whole grains, wheat bran, and high-protein foods. Persons who have sickle-cell anemia may be deficient in zinc. One interesting clinical study showed a decrease in the number of sickled red blood cells in patients who used zinc supplementation.

Nutrients	Importance
Vitamins	
Vitamin A	Deficiency is associated with anemia due to impaired hemoglobin synthesis as well as heavy menstrual bleeding.
Vitamin B_1 (thiamine)	Deficiency may cause megaloblastic (large-shaped cells) anemia.
Vitamin B_2 (riboflavin)	Aids in formation of red blood cells. Deficiency is associated with anemia.
Vitamin B_5 (pantothenic acid)	Aids in the reversal of anemia in cases with increased iron storage in the bone marrow.
Vitamin B_6 (pyridoxine)	Deficiency causes anemia.
Vitamin B_{12} (cyanocobalamin)	Essential for normal formation of blood cells. Necessary for prevention of pernicious anemia.
Folic acid (folacin)	Necessary for red blood cell formation.
Vitamin C	Aids in absorption of iron. Deficiency is associated with heavy menstrual bleeding.
Bioflavonoids	Deficiency is associated with heavy menstrual bleeding.
Vitamin E	Protects red blood cells from destruction. Important for sickle-cell anemia and anemia associated with cystic fibrosis and pancreatic insufficiency.
Minerals	
Copper	Aids in formation of red blood cells. Deficiency is associated with anemia.
Iron	Necessary for hemoglobin formation. Deficiency causes most frequent type of anemia. Can be a cause of heavy menstrual bleeding.
Zinc	May be deficient in sickle-cell anemia.
Other Factors	
Hydrochloric acid	If deficient, iron absorption is impaired. May affect iron deficiency anemia.

Herbs for Anemia & Heavy Menstrual Bleeding

Herbs can play a helpful role in your nutritional program to relieve and prevent anemia and heavy menstrual bleeding. They should be thought of as a form of extended nutrition that can be taken as either teas or capsules. Two herbs have been traditionally used to stop excessive menstrual flow and postpartum hemorrhage: golden seal and shepherd's purse. Recent research studies have supported the traditional claims made for these herbs. Golden seal contains a chemical called berberine that calms uterine muscular tension. It has also been used to calm and soothe the digestive tract. Shepherd's purse helps promote blood clotting and has also been used to help stop menstrual bleeding. If your bleeding is excessive or irregular, consult your physician. This needs to be evaluated carefully by your physician and, if necessary, medical therapy should be instituted. Excessive and irregular bleeding can be dangerous and should never be allowed to continue without medical help. For those women for whom the menstrual flow is normal but somewhat heavier than usual, the mild properties of herbs may be helpful for symptom relief.

Plants that contain bioflavonoids may also help stop and prevent heavy menstrual bleeding. Bioflavonoids help to strengthen capillaries and, along with vitamin C, can help prevent excessive bruising as well as bleeding. Bioflavonoids are found in a wide variety of fruits and flowers and are responsible for their striking colors. Good sources of bioflavonoids include citrus fruits, hawthorn berries, bilberries, cherries, and grape skins. Bioflavonoids have also been found in red clover and in some clover strains in Australia.

Other herbs help to prevent anemia by providing good sources of non-heme iron. Excellent examples are yellow dock and pau d'arco. Yellow dock is also used to help promote liver health—an important factor in decreasing heavy bleeding through regulation of excessive estrogen levels, since the liver breaks down estrogen and prepares it for excretion from the body. Tumeric, or curcumin, is also used to promote liver health in traditional medicine. Recent research suggests that it has antibacterial properties. Tumeric is a delicious herb used often for flavoring in traditional Indian dishes. Silymarin, or milk thistle, protects liver functions through its flavonoid content. These flavonoids are strong antioxidants and help protect the liver from damage. The wild yam root has been found to have the hormonal properties of progesterones. It has been used like progesterone or the progestins to help regulate the heavier menstrual bleeding found in women who are in transition into menopause.

How to Use Vitamin, Mineral, & Herbal Supplements

Good dietary habits and the use of supplements are a necessary combination for women who want to make up the nutritional deficiencies that accompany both anemia and heavy menstrual bleeding. In order to restore the level of nutrients necessary to produce an adequate number of red blood cells as well as healthy red blood cells, dietary intake may not be sufficient. Anemic women may also need to take nutrients in a concentrated supplemental form at sufficient doses to "jump start" the system into normal functioning again. This is also true for women with heavy menstrual bleeding; supplements can help reestablish a normal hormonal profile, as well as restore the strength and integrity of the capillaries and other blood vessels so that normal bleeding patterns resume.

Vitamin, mineral, and herbal supplements, however, should never be used as an excuse to continue poor dietary habits. They should be taken only with high-nutrient meals to maintain optimal health. With anemia and heavy menstrual bleeding, it is important to make sure that both your diet and your supplement program provide the extra nutrients that your body needs.

On the following pages are two formulas for nutritional supplements that you can put together yourself. These formulas are typical of those that I have used for many years with my patients. An excellent Woman's Daily Iron Nutritional System is also available through *The LifeCycles Center* described in the Appendix. (See the Appendix for specifics on ordering the product.) The Menopause Nutritional System (available through the Center) contains nutritional support for women with heavy menstrual bleeding, since this is a very common problem for women in their forties who are in transition into menopause. These prepared formulas can be used if you do not want to make up your own. I do want to emphasize, however, that any heavy menstrual bleeding problem should be evaluated by a physician. Nutritional support should not be used to replace medical therapy when heavy menstrual bleeding occurs.

Remember that all women differ somewhat in their nutritional needs. If you do take the recommended supplements for either problem, I usually recommend that you start with one-fourth to one-half of the dose recommended in this book, then slowly work your way up to a higher dosage. You may find that you feel best with slightly more or less of certain ingredients.

I recommend that all supplements be taken with meals or at least with a snack. A digestive reaction to supplements, such as nausea or indigestion, is rare. If this happens to you, stop all supplements and start them again *one at a time* until you find the offending nutrient. Any nutrient to which you have a reaction should be eliminated from your program. If you have any specific questions, ask a health-care professional who is knowledgeable about nutrition.

Optimal Nutritional Supplementation for Anemia

Vitamins and Minerals in an Herbal Base

Iron	27 mg
Vitamin C	250 mg
Vitamin E (natural d-alpha)	30 I.U.
Vitamin B complex	
B_1 (thiamine)	7.5 mg
B_2 (riboflavin)	7.5 mg
B_6 (pyridoxine)	30 mg
B_5 (pantothenic acid)	50 mg
B_3 (niacinamide)	10 mg
B_{12} (cyanocobalamin)	250 mcg
Folic acid	400 mcg
Biotin	100 mcg
Choline bitartrate	5 mg
Inositol	5 mg
PABA	5 mg
Zinc	1.5 mg
Copper	250 mcg
Betaine HCL	10 mg
Chlorophyll	35 mg
Licorice root	25 mg
Red clover	25 mg
Yellow dock	25 mg

Herbal tinctures for Anemia

Yellow dock	2 droppersful
Huckleberry	2 droppersful
Oregon grape root	2 droppersful

Optimal Nutritional Supplementation for Heavy Menstrual Bleeding

Vitamins and Minerals for Heavy Menstrual Bleeding

Vitamin A	5000 I.U.
Beta carotene (provitamin A)	5000 I.U.
Vitamin B complex	
B_1 (thiamine)	50 mg
B_2 (riboflavin)	50 mg
B_3 (niacinamide)	50 mg
B_5 (pantothenic acid)	50 mg
B_6 (pyridoxine)	30 mg
B_{12} (cyanocobalamin)	50 mcg
Folic acid	400 mcg
Biotin	200 mcg
Choline	50 mcg
Inositol	50 mg
PABA	50 mg
Vitamin C (as ascorbic acid)	1000 mg
Vitamin D	400 I.U.
Bioflavonoids	800 mg
Rutin	200 mg
Vitamin E (d-alpha tocopheryl acetate)	800 I.U.
Calcium	1200 mg
Magnesium	320 mg
Potassium	100 mg
Iron	27 mg
Zinc	15 mg
Iodine	150 mcg
Manganese	10 mg
Copper	2 mg
Selenium	25 mcg
Chromium	100 mcg
Bromelain	100 mg
Papain	65 mg
Boron	3 mg

Herbal Tinctures for Heavy Menstrual Bleeding

Tumeric	500 mg	2 Droppersful
Wild yam	500 mg	2 Droppersful
Shepherd's purse	250 mg	1 Dropperful
Golden seal	250 mg	1 Dropperful

Food Sources of Iron

Grains	Legumes	Vegetables
Bran cereal	Black beans	Brussels sprouts
(All-Bran)	Pinto beans	Spinach
Millet, dry	Garbanzo beans	Broccoli
Wheat germ	Soybeans	Sweet potatoes
Pasta, whole wheat	Kidney beans	Dandelion greens
Bran muffin	Lima beans	Green beans
Pumpernickel bread	Lentils	Corn
Oak flakes	Split peas	Leeks
Shredded wheat	Black-eyed peas	Kale
Whole wheat bread	Green peas	Swiss chard
Rye bread	Tofu	Beets
Wheat bran		Beet greens
Pearl barley		Mushrooms
White rice		Parsnips
		Carrots
(Items in each category listed from best to good)		Mustard greens
		Green pepper
		Lettuce
		Turnips
		Asparagus
		Collards
		Cauliflower
		Zucchini
		Winter squash
		Red cabbage

Food Sources of Iron

Fruits	Meat, Poultry, Seafood	Nuts and Seeds
Prune juice	Calf's liver	Sesame seeds
Figs	Beef liver	Sunflower seeds
Raisins	Chicken liver	Pistachios
Prunes, dried	Oysters	Pecans
Avocado	Trout	Sesame butter
Apple juice	Clams	Almonds
Dates, dried	Scallops	Hazelnuts (filberts)
Blackberries	Sardines	Walnuts
Pineapple	Shrimp	
Grape juice	Chicken	
Apricots, fresh	Haddock	
Cantaloupe	Cod	
Strawberries	Salmon	
Cherries		

(Items in each category listed from best to good)

Food Sources of Vitamin A		Food Sources of Vitamin B Complex (including folic acid)	
Vegetables	**Fruits**	**Vegetables**	**Meat, Poultry,**
Carrots	Apricots	**and Legumes**	**Seafood**
Carrot juice	Avocado	Alfalfa	Egg yolks*
Collard greens	Cantaloupe	Artichoke	Liver*
Dandelion	Mangoes	Asparagus	
greens	Papaya	Beets	**Grains**
Green onions	Peaches	Broccoli	Barley
Kale	Persimmons	Brussels sprouts	Bran
Parsley		Cabbage	Brown rice
Spinach	**Meat, Poultry,**	Cauliflower	Corn
Sweet potatoes	**Seafood**	Corn	Millet
Turnip greens	Crab	Garbanzo beans	Rice bran
Winter squash	Halibut	Green beans	Wheat
	Liver—all types	Kale	Wheat germ
	Mackerel	Leeks	
	Salmon	Lentils	**Sweeteners**
	Swordfish	Lima beans	Blackstrap
		Onions	molasses
		Peas	
		Pinto beans	
		Romaine lettuce	
		Soybeans	

* Eggs and meat must be from range fed, organic sources fed on non-pesticided fodder.

Food Sources of Vitamin B$_6$

Grains	Vegetables
Brown rice	Asparagus
Buckwheat flour	Beet greens
Rice bran	Broccoli
Rice polishings	Brussels sprouts
Rye flour	Cauliflower
Wheat germ	Green peas
Whole wheat	Leeks
flour	Sweet potatoes

Meat, Poultry, Seafood	Nuts and Seeds
Chicken	Sunflower
Salmon	seeds
Shrimp	
Tuna	

Food Sources of Vitamin C

Fruits	Vegetables and Legumes
Blackberries	Asparagus
Black currants	Black-eyed peas
Cantaloupe	Broccoli
Elderberries	Brussels sprouts
Grapefruit	Cabbage
Grapefruit juice	Cauliflower
Guavas	Collards
Kiwi fruit	Green onions
Mangoes	Green peas
Oranges	Kale
Orange juice	Kohlrabi
Pineapple	Parsley
Raspberries	Potatoes
Strawberries	Rutabaga
Tangerines	Sweet pepper
	Sweet potatoes
	Tomatoes
	Turnips

Meat, Poultry, Seafood
Liver—all types
Pheasant
Quail
Salmon

Food sources of Vitamin B$_{12}$

Protein
Fish
Eggs
Liver

Food Sources of Copper

Vegetables and Legumes
Kidney beans
Lentils
Lima beans
Okra
Split peas

Meat, Poultry, Seafood
Liver
Cod
Haddock
Halibut
Lobster
Oysters
Pike
Shrimp

Sweeteners
Blackstrap molasses

Fruits
Avocado
Dried figs
Prunes
Raisins

Nuts and Seeds
Almonds
Filberts
Pecans
Pistachios
Sesame seeds
Sunflower seeds
Walnuts

Food Sources of Zinc

Grains
Barley
Brown rice
Buckwheat
Corn
Cornmeal
Millet
Oatmeal
Rice bran
Rye bread
Wheat bran
Wheat germ
Wheat berries
Whole wheat bread
Whole wheat flour

Vegetables and Legumes
Black-eyed peas
Cabbage
Carrots
Garbanzo beans
Green peas
Lentils
Lettuce
Lima beans
Onions
Soy flour
Soy meal
Soy protein

Fruits
Apples
Peaches

Meat, Poultry, Seafood
Chicken
Oysters

Suggested Reading

Castleman, M. *The Healing Herbs*. Emmaus, PA: Rodale Press, 1991.

Greenwood, S., M.D. *Menopause Naturally*. Volcano, CA: Volcano Press, 1989.

Hasslering, B., S. Greenwood, M.D., and M. Castleman. *The Medical Self-Care Book of Women's Health*. New York: Doubleday, 1987.

Hogladaroom, G., R. McCorkle, and N. Woods. *The Complete Book of Women's Health*. Englewood Cliffs, NJ: Prentice Hall, 1982.

Kirschmann, J., and L. Dunne. *Nutrition Almanac*. New York: McGraw-Hill, 1984.

Kutsky, R. *Vitamins and Hormones*. New York: Van Nostrand Reinhold, 1973.

Lark, S., M.D. *Menopause Self-Help Book*. Berkeley, CA: Celestial Arts, 1990.

Lark, S., M.D. *Premenstrual Syndrome Self-Help Book*. Berkeley, CA: Celestial Arts, 1984.

Mowrey, D., Ph.D. *The Scientific Validation of Herbal Medicine*. New Canaan, CT: Keats Publishing, 1986.

Murray, M., N.D. *The 21st Century Herbal*. Bellevue, WA: Vita-Line, Inc.

Padus, E. *The Woman's Encyclopedia of Health and Natural Healing*. Emmaus, PA: Rodale Press, 1981.

Reuben, C., and J. Priestly. *Essential Supplements for Women*. New York: Perigree Books, 1988.

Articles

Ajayi, O. A., et al. Hematological response to supplements of riboflavin and ascorbic acid in Nigerian young adults. *European Journal of Hematology* 1990; 44:209-212.

Beard, J. L., et al. Impaired thermoregulations and thyroid function in iron-deficiency anemia. *American Journal of Clinical Nutrition* 1990; 52:813-9.

Bernat, I. Iron deficiency. *Iron Metabolism*. New York, Plenum Press, 1983: 215-74.

Bernat, I. Pyridoxine responsive anemia. *Iron Metabolism*. New York, Plenum Press, 1983; 313-14.

Brewer G. J., et al. Suppression of irreversibly sickled erythrocytes by zinc therapy in sickle cell anemia. *Journal of Laboratory and Clinical Medicine* 1977; 90(3):549-54.

Cheng, E. W., et al. Estrogenic activity of some naturally occurring isoflavones. *Annals of New York Academy of Sciences* 1955; 61(3):652.

Clemetson, C. A. B., et al. Capillary strength and the menstrual cycle. *New York Academy of Sciences* 1962; 93(7):277.

Cohen, J. D., and H. W. Rubin. Functional menorrhagia: Treatment with bioflavonoids and vitamin C. *Current Therapeutic Research* 1960; 2(11):539.

Corash, L., et al. Reduced chronic hemolysis during high-dose vitamin E administration in Mediterranean type glucose-6-phosphate dehydrogenase deficiency. *New England Journal of Medicine* 1980; 303:416-20.

Drake, J. R., and C. D. Fitch. Status of vitamin E as an erythropoietic factor. *American Journal of Clinical Nutrition* 1980; 33:2386-93.

Dunlap W. M., et al. Anemia and neutropenia caused by copper deficiency. *Annals of Internal Medicine* 1974; 80:470.

Farley, P., M.D., and J. Foland, M.D. Iron deficiency anemia: How to diagnose and correct. *Postgraduate Medicine* 1990; 87(2):89-101.

Farrell, P. M., et al. *Journal of Clinical Investigation* 1970; 60:233-41.

Harris, C. The vicious cycle of anemia and menorrhagia. *Canadian Medical Association Journal* 1957; 77:98.

Hines, J. D., and D. Love. Abnormal vitamin B6 metabolism in sideroblastic anemia: Effect of pyridoxal phosphate therapy. *Clinical Research* 1975; 23:403A.

Hines, J. D., and J. W. Harris. Pyridoxine-responsive anemia: Description of three patients with megaloblastic erythopoiesis. *American Journal of Clinical Nutrition* 1964; 14:137-46.

Hodges, R. E., et al. Hematopoietic studies in vitamin A deficiency. *American Journal of Clinical Nutrition* 1978; 31:876-85.

Hunt, J. R., et al. Ascorbic acid: Effect on ongoing iron absorption and status in iron-depleted young women. *American Journal of Clinical Nutrition* 1990; 51:649-55.

Izak, G., et al. *Scandinavian Journal of Haematology* 1973; 11:236.

Jacobs, P., et al. Gastric acidity and iron absorption. *British Journal of Haematology* 1966; 12:728-36.

Jacobs, P., et al. Role of hydrochloric acid in iron absorption. *Journal of Applied Physiology* 1964; 19(2):187-8.

Kark, J. A., et al. Pyridoxal phosphate as an antisickling agent in vitro. *Journal of Clinical Investigation* 1983; 71:1224.

Lane, M., and C. P. Alfrey, Jr. The anemia of human riboflavin deficiency. *Blood* 1965; 25(4):432-42.

Leonard, P. J., and M. S. Losowsky. Effect of alpha-tocopherol administration on red cell survival in vitamin E-deficient human subjects. *American Journal of Clinical Nutrition* 1971; 24:388-93.

Lindenbaum, J., et al. *New England Journal of Medicine* 1963; 269:875.

Lithgow, P. M. and W. M. Politzer. Vitamin A in the treatment of menorrhagia. *South African Medical Journal* 1977; 51:191.

Mangel, H., et al. Thiamine-dependent beriberi in the "thiamine-responsive anemia syndrome." *New England Journal of Medicine* 1984; 311:836-8.

McCurdy, P. R. Is there an anemia responsive to pantothenic acid? *Journal of American Geriatric Society* 1973; 21(2):88-91.

Mejia, L., and F. Chew. Hematologic effect of supplementing anemic children with vitamin A alone and in combination with iron. *American Journal of Clinical Nutrition* 1988; 48:595-600.

Monsen, E. R. Ascorbic acid: An enhancing factor in iron absorption. In *Nutritional Bioavailability of Iron*. American Chemical Society, 1982, pp. 85-95.

Natta, C. L., and L. Machlin. Plasma levels of tocopherol in sickle cell anemia subjects. *American Journal of Clinical Nutrition* 1979; 32:1359.

Natta, C. L., and R. D. Reynolds. Apparent vitamin B6 deficiency in sickle cell anemia. *American Journal of Clinical Nutrition* 1984; 40:235-9.

Natta, C. L., et al. A decrease in irreversibly sickled erythrocytes in sickle cell anemia patients given vitamin E. *American Journal of Clinical Nutrition* 1980; 33:968-71.

Niell, H. B., et al. Zinc metabolism in sickle cell anemia. Journal of the *American Medical Association* 1979; 242 (24):2686-90.

Pearse, H. A., and J. D. Trisler. A rational approach to the treatment of habitual abortion and menometorrhagia. *Clinical Medicine* 1957; 9:1081.

Penrod, J. C., et al. Impact on iron status of introducing cow's milk in the second six months of life. *Journal of Pediatric Gastroenterology and Nutrition* 1990; 10:462-467.

Pierce, L. E., and C. E. Rath. Evidence for folic acid deficiency in the genesis of anemic sickle cell crisis. *Blood* 1962; 20:19.

Pope, G. S., et al. Isolation of an oestrogenic isoflavone (biochanin A) from red clover. *Chemistry and Industry* 1953; 10:1042.

Porter, K. G., et al. Anemia and low serum copper during zinc therapy. *Lancet* October 8, 1977; 774.

Preuter, G. W. A treatment for excessive uterine bleeding. *Applied Therapeutics* 1961; 5:351.

Rogers, L. E., et al. Thiamine-responsive megaloblastic anemia. *Journal of Pediatrics* 1969; 74(4):494-504.

Sood, S. K., et al. *Journal of Tropical Medicine and Hygiene* 1974; 77:177.

Tant, D. Megaloblastic anemia due to pyridoxine deficiency associated with prolonged ingestion of an estrogen-containing oral contraceptive. *British Medical Journal* October 23, 1976; 979.

Taylor, F. A. Habitual abortion: therapeutic evaluation of citrus bioflavonoids. *Western Journal of Surgery, Obstetrics and Gynecology* 1956; 5:280.

Taymor, M. L., et al. The etiological role of chronic iron deficiency in production of menorrhagia. *Journal of the American Medical Association* 1964; 187:323.

Taymor, M. L., et al. Menorrhagia due to chronic iron deficiency. *Obstetrics and Gynecology* 1960; 16:571.

Viana, M. B., and R. I. Carvalho. Thiamine-responsive megaloblastic anemia sensorineural deafness and diabetes mellitus: A new syndrome? *Journal of Pediatrics* 1978; 93:235.

Williams, D. M. Copper deficiency in humans. *Seminars in Hematology* 1983; 20(2):118-28.

6

Dietary Principles for Anemia & Heavy Menstrual Flow

$\mathcal{G}$ood nutrition is absolutely essential for women with anemia and heavy menstrual bleeding. Medical studies have shown that poor nutritional habits can aggravate both of these problems. A diet full of high-stress foods such as fat, sugar, chocolate, alcohol, and caffeine does not provide the nutrients you need for healing and repair and can actually worsen the symptoms of bleeding and anemia. In contrast, a healthful and well-chosen diet can make a tremendous difference in preventing debilitating symptoms. Both anemia and heavy menstrual bleeding can be prevented and controlled, at least in part, by proper nutrition. A healthful diet includes foods such as fresh fruits and vegetables, whole grains, beans, seeds and nuts, high-quality vegetable oils, and small amounts of fish and poultry. These high-nutrient foods, together with appropriate supplements, are absolutely necessary to promote optimal health and well-being. Proper food selection is an essential part of your self-help program. In this chapter, I provide the information you need about the best foods to prevent anemia and heavy menstrual bleeding, as well as which foods to avoid.

Foods that Help Treat or Prevent Anemia & Heavy Menstrual Bleeding

You should emphasize the following foods in your diet. These foods will also help the healing process proceed in the fastest and most efficient manner, since they contain the building blocks that your body needs for repair.

Whole Grains. Grains are an excellent source of iron for anemic women and for women who have depleted iron stores due to excessive menstrual bleeding. The best grain sources of iron include whole grains such as millet, barley, rye, whole wheat, oats, and brown rice. Enriched grain products such as noodles, macaroni, and white rice provide additional sources of iron. Grains and other vegetarian iron sources contain non-heme iron, which is unlike the iron found in meat. Non-heme iron is poorly absorbed from the digestive tract, with an absorption rate of approximately 5 percent. In contrast, the iron from meat and eggs is absorbed five times more efficiently. Non-heme iron is also susceptible to blocking agents, such as the tannin found in tea and the calcium in antacids. Food preservatives can further decrease iron absorption.

However, absorption of non-heme iron can be facilitated by taking at least 75 milligrams of vitamin C per meal. This can be accomplished easily in planning meals that combine grains with fruits and vegetables. At breakfast you can increase iron absorption by adding strawberries to your corn flakes or oatmeal, or by eating a fresh orange or grapefruit. At dinner you can eat pasta or rice with vegetables like broccoli, brussels sprouts, cauliflower, or green pepper to facilitate iron absorption.

Whole grains have many other benefits, too. They are high in fiber, the indigestible part of plant food. Fiber is very helpful in relieving constipation as well as preventing other digestive problems such as hiatus hernia and diverticulitis. Cancer of the colon, breast, uterus, and ovaries have been linked to a high-fat diet. A diet high in saturated fats should be avoided at all cost. Whole grains appear to help bind fat and remove it from the body, as well as help to control cholesterol. Oat and rice bran are particularly useful in achieving these results. Grains are also an excellent source of protein, particularly when combined with beans and peas. They are an excellent source of B-complex vitamins, vitamin E, and various minerals, all of which are needed for both normal production and survival of red blood cells.

I generally recommend that women use whole grains and whole grain flour instead of the refined grain products for their higher nutrient and fiber content. Many women with anemia and heavy menstrual bleeding also complain of poor digestive function. If this is true for you, I recommend emphasizing all grains except whole wheat. Wheat contains a protein called gluten, which is difficult to digest and can be highly allergenic. I have seen wheat increase symptoms such as fatigue, depression, and bloating in many of my women patients.

A wide range of whole grain products and whole grain flours is available today, including cereals, breads, crackers, pancakes, and pasta. The following choices can be prepared and eaten in a variety of ways.

Whole Grain Cereals. Puffed millet, unsweetened granola, puffed corn, and puffed rice are available as cold breakfast cereals. Cream of rye and buckwheat groats are also good sources of iron. These products can be found in health food stores. Your best bet if you shop in a supermarket is the slow-cooking, old-fashioned Quaker Oats (the quick-cooking kind is a refined grain product and should be avoided). Health food stores offer a wider choice of iron-rich cereals.

Whole Grain Breads. Many different whole grain breads are available at health food stores. Examples include breads made of rice, sesame and millet, oatmeal, soy and potato, rye, and lima beans. Choose brands made without added sugar.

Crackers. Both rye and rice crackers are available in supermarkets. Rye flour, in particular, is a good source of iron. Crackers can be used for snacks or open-faced sandwiches.

Brown rice cakes are particularly good with soy spreads, tuna salad, or fruit and nut spreads.

Pancakes. Pancakes can be made with buckwheat, rice flour, or triticale. Concentrated forms of sweeteners such as maple syrup, honey, molasses, and applesauce can be used in small amounts.

Pasta. Pasta made from buckwheat, rice, corn, and soybeans are readily available in health food and ethnic food stores. These provide good sources of iron, as do enriched noodles and spaghetti.

Legumes. Beans and peas are excellent sources of iron. I especially recommend black beans, pinto beans, kidney beans, chickpeas, lentils, lima beans, and soybean products for women with anemia and heavy menstrual bleeding. These foods are particularly high in iron and tend to be good sources of copper and zinc. Legumes are very high in B-complex vitamins, folic acid, and vitamin B_6, all necessary nutrients for treating anemia. Legumes are also excellent sources of protein and provide all the essential amino acids when eaten with grains. (Good examples of grain and legume combinations include meals such as beans and rice, or cornbread and lentil soup.) Sufficient protein intake is important for healthy red blood cell development, and legumes provide an excellent, easily utilized source.

As with grains, legumes are an excellent source of fiber and can help digestive function. They digest slowly and can help regulate the blood sugar level, a trait they share with whole grains. As a result, legumes are an excellent food for women with diabetes or blood sugar imbalances. Some women find that gas is a problem when they eat beans. Gas can be minimized by eating beans in small amounts or by using digestive enzymes such as papain and bromelain (derived from plants) or pancreatin capsules, which are similar to the enzymes found in the human pancreas.

Vegetables. These are particularly good foods for both anemia and heavy menstrual bleeding since they are extremely high in both vitamin and mineral content. Vegetables high in vitamin A have bright and attractive colors, such as yellow, red, orange, and intense green. They include sweet potatoes, carrots, squash, peppers, kale, and lettuce, as well as many other common foods. Vitamin A is a very important nutrient for the prevention of heavy menstrual bleeding; a deficiency puts you at higher risk of cervical cancer. Vitamin A is also needed for normal red blood cell production. The type of vitamin A found in vegetables is water soluble and does not accumulate in toxic levels in the body. For this reason, vegetables high in vitamin A content can be eaten in large amounts.

Many vegetables are high in vitamin C. Vitamin C, along with bioflavonoids, helps prevent and can actually help stop excessive bleeding. It also helps women absorb iron more efficiently when foods containing both nutrients are eaten together. Like vitamin A, it seems to protect women from developing cervical cancer. Vitamin C is also important for immune function, wound healing, and stress. Vegetables high in vitamin C include broccoli, brussels sprouts, cauliflower, kale, parsley, peppers, peas, tomatoes, and potatoes. As you can see, there are many good vegetable sources for this nutrient.

Many vegetables contain high amounts of iron. Some of the best include beet greens, swiss chard, potatoes, mushrooms, tomatoes, spinach, brussels sprouts, sweet potatoes, broccoli, kale, and green beans. These vegetables are also good sources of other minerals, such as calcium, magnesium, and potassium. I always recommend that women eat vegetables raw or steamed to preserve the nutrient value. Be careful not to boil or overcook, because important vitamins and minerals can be lost in the cooking process.

Fruits. Fruits provide a wide range of vitamins and minerals. Fruits are a terrific source of vitamins A and C, both of which help prevent and relieve heavy menstrual bleeding and anemia. Most whole fruits contain some vitamin C, with berries, oranges, grapefruits, and melons being excellent sources of this essential nutrient. Fruits that are orange and yellow in color, such as apricots, tangerines, papayas, and persimmons, are excellent sources of vitamin A.

Fresh and dried fruits are an excellent dietary substitute for cookies, candies, cakes, and other foods high in refined sugar. Whole fruit is also a healthful snack; it is beneficial for your body because of its high fiber content. Even though fruit is high in sugar, its high-fiber content helps slow down absorption of the sugar into the blood and thereby helps stabilize the blood sugar level. The fiber content in fruit also helps prevent constipation. I recommend, however, using fruit juices in small quantities. Fruit juice does not contain the bulk or fiber of the whole fruit. As a result, it acts more like table sugar and can destabilize your blood sugar level in a dramatic manner if used to excess. In the case of fruit juice, less is better. If you want to have fruit juice on a frequent basis, mix it half-and-half with water.

Seeds and Nuts. Seeds and nuts are good sources of non-heme or vegetarian iron. Particularly useful are sesame seeds, sunflower seeds, pistachios, pecans, and almonds. They are also very high in other essential nutrients that women need, such as magnesium, calcium, and fatty acids. Because seeds and nuts are very high in calories, they should be eaten in small amounts.

The oils in seeds and nuts are very perishable, so exposure to light, heat, and oxygen should be avoided. Seeds and nuts should be eaten raw and unsalted to get the benefit of their essential fatty acids—which are good for your skin and hair—as well as to avoid the negative effects of too much salt. Whenever possible, purchase unshelled nuts and seeds. If you buy them already shelled, refrigerate them so their oils don't become rancid. Do not buy broken nuts as they become rancid faster and lose their nutrient value. Nuts and seeds make a wonderful garnish on salads, vegetable dishes, and casseroles. They can also be eaten as a main source of protein with snacks and light meals.

Meat, Poultry, and Seafood. Meat is an exceptionally good source of the easily absorbed heme iron. It also contains high levels of other essential nutrients needed to prevent anemia, especially vitamin C, vitamin B_{12}, and folic acid. Meat is also high in other blood builders, including protein, copper, and zinc. Your best meat choices include liver, oysters, trout, scallops, shrimp, poultry, and venison.

If you are deficient in hydrochloric acid and find meat difficult to digest, you may need to use a small amount of hydrochloric acid as a digestive supplement with meat-containing meals. You can find digestive enzymes in a health food store.

If you do include meat in your anemia and heavy menstrual bleeding dietary program, I recommend that you use it in very small amounts (3 ounces or less per day). Most Americans eat much more protein than is healthy in their diets. Excessive amounts of protein are difficult to digest and stress the kidneys. Except for fish, meat is also a primary source of unhealthy saturated fats which put you at higher risk for heart disease and cancer. Instead of using meat as your only source of protein, I recommend that you increase your intake of grains, beans, and raw seeds and nuts, which contain protein as well as many other important nutrients. For many years I have recommended that my patients use meat more as a garnish and a flavoring for casseroles, stir-fries, and soups. I also recommend buying organic, range-fed meat—the animal's exposure to pesticides, antibiotics, and hormones is reduced.

Oils. Certain oils, including wheat germ oil, soybean oil, and corn oil, contain vitamin E, which is an important nutrient for red blood cell survival. For women who are in transition into menopause, oils with high vitamin E content have the additional benefit of helping to suppress hot flashes and menopause-related moodiness. Wheat germ oil contains the highest levels of vitamin E and, in fact, is the source for most natural vitamin E sold on the market today. Cold-pressed oils tend to be fresher and purer. Keep oils refrigerated to avoid rancidity. Vegetable oils, such as olive oil and sesame oil, can be used in small amounts for cooking, stir-frying, and sautéing.

Oils such as flax oil or pumpkin seed oil should not be used for cooking since they are heat sensitive and are altered chemically at high temperatures.

Foods to Avoid with Anemia & Heavy Menstrual Bleeding

The following foods should be avoided or at least limited in your diet. These foods can increase the tendency toward both anemia and heavy menstrual bleeding. You will notice that many of these foods are recognized as being stressful and unhealthy for your body in general.

Dairy Products. Women with anemia and heavy menstrual bleeding should avoid dairy products. Clinical studies have shown that dairy products decrease iron absorption in anemic women. Their high saturated fat content is a risk factor for promoting excess estrogen levels in the body, a common cause of heavy menstrual bleeding. And this isn't the only bad news. Dairy products have many other unhealthy effects on a woman's body. The tryptophan in milk has a sedative effect that increases fatigue, a real problem for anemic women. Many women are allergic to dairy products or lack the enzymes to digest milk, resulting in digestive problems such as bloating, gas, and bowel changes. Intolerance to dairy products can hamper the absorption and assimilation of the calcium they contain. Dairy products are also high in salt, which can increase bloating and increase the risk of high blood pressure, heart attacks, and strokes.

Women who are concerned about their calcium intake can turn to the many other good dietary sources of this essential nutrient. These include beans, peas, soybeans, sesame seeds, soup stock made from chicken or fish bones, and green leafy vegetables. For food preparation, soy milk, potato milk, and nut milk are excellent substitutes for cow's milk. Nondairy milks are readily available at health food stores. You can also use a supplement containing calcium, magnesium, and vitamin D to make sure your intake is sufficient.

Fats. Fat constitutes 40 percent of the calories in the typical American diet. Most of this fat comes from unhealthy saturated sources such as dairy products, red meat, and eggs. This diet tends to promote heavy menstrual bleeding in susceptible women, because excessive saturated fat intake is stressful to the liver and helps to increase excess estrogen levels. This type of fat also puts women at high risk for heart disease and cancer of the breast, uterus, and ovaries. Women on a high-fat diet also tend to accumulate excess weight more easily. Eat more fruits, vegetables, grains, fish, and poultry instead of foods high in saturated fats. As often as possible, eat fresh and homemade foods prepared with a minimum of fats and oils. If you must eat packaged and processed foods, read the labels and avoid those foods with a high fat content. Red meat should be used only in small amounts. Avoid rich recipes that use large amounts of butter, cream, cheese, or other high-fat foods in the preparation. Instead, flavor foods with garlic, onions, herbs, lemon juice, or a little olive oil (a monosaturated fat that doesn't increase your cholesterol level). Eat raw seeds and nuts rather than cooked ones (cooking alters the nature of the oils), and use them sparingly because of their high fat content.

Alcohol. Alcohol should be avoided entirely or consumed only in small amounts by women with anemia and heavy menstrual bleeding. Alcohol depletes the body's B-complex vitamins and minerals, which can worsen anemia. It also disrupts carbohydrate metabolism. Alcohol is toxic to the liver and can affect the liver's ability to metabolize hormones efficiently. Excessive alcohol intake has been associated with lack of ovulation and elevated estrogen levels, which can trigger heavy menstrual bleeding in susceptible women. In large amounts, alcohol can be toxic to the heart and nervous system. When used carefully, not exceeding 4 ounces of wine per day, 10 ounces of beer, or 1 ounce of hard liquor, it can have a delightfully relaxing effect. It makes us more sociable and enhances the taste of food. For optimal health, however, I recommend using alcohol only as an occasional treat, not more than once or twice a week.

Women who are particularly susceptible to the negative effects of alcohol shouldn't drink it at all.

If you entertain often and enjoy social drinking, I recommend that you try nonalcoholic beverages. A nonalcoholic cocktail, such as mineral water with a twist of lime or lemon or a dash of bitters, is a good substitute. "Near beer" is a nonalcoholic beer substitute that tastes quite good. Light wine and beer have a lower alcohol content than hard liquor, liqueurs, and regular wine.

Caffeine. Coffee, black tea, soft drinks, and chocolate—all of these foods contain caffeine, a stimulant that many women use to increase their energy level and alertness and to decrease fatigue. Unfortunately, caffeine has many negative effects on the body. Caffeine used in excess also increases anxiety, irritability, and mood swings. This can be a real problem for women with anemia who have lowered emotional and physical reserves. Caffeine also depletes the body's stores of B-complex vitamins. This interferes with carbohydrate metabolism and healthy liver function, which helps to regulate estrogen levels and menstrual bleeding. Many menopausal women also complain that caffeine increases the frequency of hot flashes. Coffee, black tea, chocolate, and soft drinks all act to inhibit iron absorption. Black tea contains tannins that inhibit iron absorption, particularly when a meal is deficient in vitamin C. Polyphenols found in coffee also interfere with iron absorption, as do the oxalic acid found in chocolate and the additives in soft drinks. All of these foods should be avoided by a woman with anemia.

Considering all of these negative effects, women should either cut down dramatically on caffeine intake or eliminate it entirely. Because cutting out caffeine can cause withdrawal symptoms such as irritability and headaches, I recommend that women eliminate caffeine gradually. To start, mix half a cup of regular coffee with half a cup of decaffeinated coffee. I recommend using water-processed decaffeinated coffee, which is extracted with hot water rather than chemicals. After a month or two on decaffeinated coffee, switch to grain-based coffee substitutes, such as Pero, Postum, or Caffix. Because they have a calming effect, herbal teas made from chamomile and hops can actually be therapeutic for women with anxiety.

Sugar.   Like alcohol, sugar depletes the body's B-complex vitamins and minerals, which can increase nervous tension and anxiety (real problems for anemic women). Unfortunately, most Americans eat too much sugar—the average American eats 120 pounds per year. Sugar addiction is very common in our society in people of all ages. Many people use sweet foods as a way to deal with their frustrations and other upsets. Many convenience foods, including salad dressing, catsup, and relish, contain high levels of both sugar and salt. Sugar is the main ingredient in soft drinks and in desserts such as candies, cookies, cakes, and ice cream. Foods high in sugar content also lead to tooth loss through tooth decay and gum disease. Of even greater significance is the fact that excessive sugar intake can have a negative effect on diabetes and blood sugar imbalances.

Try to satisfy your sweet tooth instead with healthier foods, such as fruit or grain-based desserts like oatmeal cookies sweetened with fruit or honey. You will find that small amounts of these foods can satisfy your cravings. Instead of disrupting your mood and energy level, they actually have a healthful and balancing effect.

Salt.   While not directly contributing to anemia and heavy menstrual bleeding, excessive salt intake should be avoided. Too much dietary salt can increase high blood pressure, bloating, and fluid retention, and can contribute to osteoporosis in menopausal women. Unfortunately, large amounts of salt are commonly found in the American diet as table salt (sodium chloride), MSG (monosodium glutamate), and a variety of food additives. Fast foods such as hamburgers, hot dogs, french fries, pizza, and tacos are loaded with salt and saturated fats. Common processed foods such as soups, potato chips, cheese, olives, salad dressings, and catsup (to name only a few) are also very high in salt. To make matters worse, many people add too much salt while cooking and seasoning their meals.

For women of all ages, I recommend eliminating added salt in your meals. For flavor, use seasonings like garlic, herbs, spices, and lemon juice. Avoid processed foods that are high in salt, including canned foods, olives, pickles, potato chips, tortilla chips, catsup, and salad dressings. Many frozen entrees are also too high in salt and fat content. Learn to read labels and look for the word sodium (salt). If it appears high on the list of ingredients, don't buy the product. Many items in health food stores are labeled "no salt added." Some supermarkets offer "no added salt" foods in their diet or health food sections.

Substitute Healthy Ingredients in Recipes

Over the years of working in nutritional medicine, I have found it easy to adapt many "forbidden recipes" to the needs of my own nutritional program. These high-stress recipes would start out filled with ingredients I couldn't normally eat—fats, dairy products, chocolate, and sugar. By eliminating the high-stress ingredients and replacing them with healthier, more nutritious substitutes, I could still make almost any recipe in my files. I have recommended this technique for years to my patients, who are delighted to find that they can still have their favorite dishes, but in much healthier versions. This is particularly important for women with anemia and heavy menstrual bleeding, since proper dietary intake can play a major role in the healing process.

One method of modifying your diet is to totally eliminate the chocolate, milk products, sugar, salt, and other high-stress ingredients that many recipes call for. These items are not necessary to make foods taste good, and they can worsen your symptoms. If you want to retain a high-stress ingredient, you can substantially reduce the amount you use, and still retain the flavor and taste. Most of us have palates jaded by too much salt, fat, sugar, and other flavorings. In many dishes, we taste only the additives; we never really enjoy the delicious flavor of the foods themselves. Now that I make a habit of substituting low-stress ingredients in my cooking, I find that I enjoy the subtle taste of the dishes much more. Also, I find that my health and vitality continue to improve with the deletion of high-stress ingredients from my food. The following information tells you how to substitute healthy ingredients in your own recipes. The substitutions are simple to make and should benefit your health greatly.

How to Substitute for Dairy Products

Use soy cheese in food preparation and cooking. Soy cheese is an excellent substitute for cow's milk cheese. It is lower in fat and salt, and the fat that it contains isn't saturated. There are many brands available in health food stores, as well as many different flavors—mozzarella, cheddar, American, and jack. The quality of these products keeps improving all the time. You can use soy cheese as a perfect cheese substitute in sandwiches, salads, pizzas, lasagnas, and casseroles.

Decrease the amount of cow's milk cheese you use in food preparation and cooking. If you must use cow's milk cheese in cooking, decrease the amount by one-half to two-thirds so that it becomes a flavoring or garnish, rather than a major source of fat and protein. Soft tofu can be added to the recipes to replace the volume of cheese you have omitted. I have done this often with lasagna, layering the lasagna noodles with tofu and topping with melted soy cheese for a delicious dish. The tofu, which is bland, takes on the taste of the tomato sauce. If you cannot give up cow's milk products, try to use the lower-fat cheese now available. Goat's or sheep's milk cheese in small amounts can also be used to replace cow's milk cheese, since the fat they contain is more easily emulsified in the body.

Milk can often be easily replaced in recipes. Substitute potato milk, soy milk, nut milk, or grain milk for cow's milk. Soy milk and nut milk are available at most health food stores. Soy milk is particularly good and comes in many flavors. Many nondairy milks are good sources of calcium and can be used for drinking, eating, or baking. (See Chapter 7 for an easy way to make an almond-based milk substitute.) One of my personal favorites is a nondairy milk that is made from an all-vegetable potato base. It is creamy and sweet and tastes very similar to the best cow's milk, with none of the unhealthy characteristics of dairy products. Even my 10-year-old daughter likes it. The potato-based milk is high in calcium and can be bought dry so that you can store it. It mixes easily in water and can be used exactly as you use cow's milk for beverages, cooking, and baking. Potato milk is available through *The LIFECYCLES Center*.

Substitute flax oil for butter. Flax oil is the best substitute for butter that I have found. It is a golden, rich oil that looks and tastes quite a bit like butter. It is delicious on anything you would normally top with butter—toast, rice, popcorn, steamed vegetables, and potatoes. Flax oil is extremely high in essential fatty acids—the type of fat that is very healthy for a woman's body. Essential fatty acids help promote normal hormonal function. Flax oil is quite perishable, however, because it is sensitive to heat and light. You cannot cook with it—cook the food first and add the flax oil before serving. It also needs to be refrigerated. There are so many health benefits to flax oil that I recommend it highly. You can find it in health food stores or order it from *The LIFECYCLES Center* if there is no health food store near you.

How to Substitute for Caffeinated Foods and Beverages

Drink substitutes for coffee and black tea. For cooking, try the grain-based coffee substitutes, such as Pero, Postum, and Caffix.

Use decaffeinated coffee or tea as a transition beverage. For women who cannot give up coffee, start by substituting water-processed decaffeinated coffee for the real thing. Then try to wean yourself from coffee altogether, or drink a coffee substitute.

Use herbal teas for energy and vitality. Many women drink coffee simply for the pick-up they get from it. Their cups of coffee in the morning enable them to wake up and function through the day. Use ginger instead. It is a great herbal stimulant that won't wreck your health. See recipe section for instructions on how to make ginger tea.

Substitute carob for chocolate. Unsweetened carob tastes like chocolate but is far more nutritious. A member of the legume family, carob is high in calcium. It can be purchased in chunk form as a substitute for chocolate candy, or as a powder to be used in baking or drinks. Be careful, however, not to overindulge; carob, like chocolate, is high in calories and fat. It should be considered a treat and a cooking aid to be used only in small amounts.

How to Substitute for Sugar

Cut the amount of sweetener in your recipes by one-third to one-half. Americans tend to be addicted to sugar. Most of us grew up on highly sugared soft drinks, candy, and rich pastries—no wonder the incidence of diabetes is soaring among our population. I have found that as women decrease their sugar intake, most of them begin to really enjoy the subtle flavors of the foods they eat.

Substitute more concentrated sweeteners. Concentrated sweeteners such as honey and maple syrup have a sweeter taste per quantity used than table sugar. Using these substitutes will allow you to decrease the actual amount of sweetener in a recipe. If you use a concentrated sweetener in place of sugar in an ordinary recipe, reduce the liquid content in the recipe by one-fourth cup. If no liquid is used in the recipe, add 3 to 5 tablespoons of flour for each three-fourths cup of concentrated sweetener.

Substitute fruit for sugar in pastries. In making muffins and cookies, you may want to try deleting sugar altogether and adding extra fruits and nuts.

How to Substitute for Salt

Substitute potassium-based products for table salt (sodium chloride). Potassium-based products are much healthier and will not aggravate heart disease or hypertension.

Use powdered seaweeds such as kelp or nori to season vegetables, grains, and salads. They are high in essential iodine and trace elements.

Use herbs instead of salt for flavoring. Their flavors are much more subtle and will help even the most jaded palate appreciate the taste of fresh fruits, vegetables, and meats.

Use liquid flavoring agents with advertised low-sodium content. Low-salt soy sauce and Bragg's Amino Acids, a liquid soybean-based flavoring agent, are delicious when used as salt substitutes in cooking. Add them to soups, casseroles, stir-fries, and other dishes at the end of the cooking process. You will find that you need only a small amount for intense flavoring.

How to Substitute for White Flour (Wheat Based)

Use whole grain, nonwheat flour. White flour loses most of its nutrient content through processing. Substitute whole grain flour, which is much higher in essential nutrients, including the B-complex vitamins and many minerals. It is also higher in fiber content.

Use rice flour or barley flour as a wheat substitute. Rice flour makes excellent cookies, cakes, and other pastries. Barley flour is best used for pie crusts.

How to Substitute for Alcohol

Use low-alcohol or nonalcoholic products for cooking. Substitute low-alcohol or nonalcoholic wine or beer when cooking or preparing sauces and marinades. Much of the flavor that alcohol imparts will be retained, and the stress factor will decrease substantially.

Substitutes for Common High-Stress Ingredients

3/4 cup sugar	1/2 cup honey
	1/4 cup molasses
	1/2 cup maple syrup
	1/2 ounce barley malt
	1 cup apple butter
	2 cups apple juice
1 cup milk	1 cup soy, potato, nut, or grain milk
1 tablespoon butter	1 tablespoon flax oil (must be used raw and unheated)
1/2 teaspoon salt	1 tablespoon miso
	1/2 teaspoon potassium chloride salt substitute
	1/2 teaspoon Mrs. Dash, Spike
	1/2 teaspoon herbs (basil, tarragon, oregano, etc.)
1-1/2 cups cocoa	1 cup powdered carob
1 square chocolate	3/4 tablespoon powdered carob
1 tablespoon coffee	1 tablespoon decaffeinated coffee
	1 tablespoon Pero, Postum, Caffix, or other grain-based coffee substitute
4 ounces wine	4 ounces light wine
8 ounces beer	8 ounces near beer
1 cup white flour (wheat based)	1 cup barley flour (pie crust)
	1 cup rice flour (cookies, cakes, breads)

7

Menus, Meal Plans, & Recipes

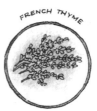
FRENCH THYME

$\mathcal{M}$any of my patients with anemia and heavy menstrual bleeding have asked me for specific recipes and meal plans to help optimize their healing program. Unfortunately, there are very few of these specific resources available for women. For instance, no cookbooks adequately address a woman's needs for specific nutrients. Most cookbooks have dishes that look and taste great but are laden with ingredients that can actually worsen a woman's condition—including such high-stress foods as dairy products, fats, chocolate, sugar, and caffeinated beverages. Some recent cookbooks do present low-calorie "light dishes." Although these cookbooks eliminate fats and sugars from the recipes, they still don't give women with anemia and heavy menstrual bleeding the therapeutic levels of specific nutrients they require.

To answer this need, I have developed a number of meal plans and recipes specifically for women with anemia and heavy menstrual bleeding. Not only have the recipes been designed to look and taste good, but they contain high levels of the nutrients you need to help rebuild and repair your body as well as those needed to help prevent anemia and heavy menstrual bleeding.

I have truly found, in my two decades as a physician, that

food is therapy. The right dietary program can have a major impact on how quickly you heal. I often tell my patients that since we all must eat, we might as well be nourishing ourselves with foods that help us stay optimally healthy. I have rarely found a woman who disagrees with this logic. Once your body begins to become healthier, it will become apparent to you that food plays a major role in promoting and maintaining female health.

I learned of the great benefits a healthy diet can bring when I permanently changed my dietary habits in my late twenties. To treat a severe case of PMS and menstrual cramps that had been plaguing me for years, I decided to change my eating habits. My health problems cleared up beautifully when I made the necessary nutritional changes. I am as healthy now in my late forties as I was in my twenties, in part because I eat a healthy and nutrient-rich diet. The past 20 years have been a real adventure. I have tried many new foods and developed many recipes to meet the needs of my own body and those of my patients.

The recipes I've included in this chapter are quick and easy to prepare. Most women have very busy lives, and I have found that anything too complicated won't work for me or my patients. Best of all, these recipes are delicious and satisfying as well as healthful. I hope that you enjoy them as much as I do.

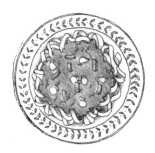

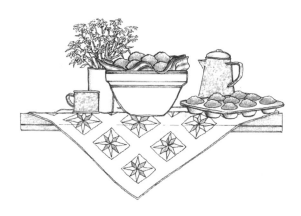

Menus

Breakfast

These easy-to-prepare menus will provide a variety of healthful and delicious meals. They can also act as guidelines as you create your own meal plans. I have developed them for their content of the essential nutrients that help to build healthy red blood cells. Starred (*) recipes are included in the following section.

Flax cereal with raisins*
Roasted grain beverage
(coffee substitute)

Flax shake*
Prunes

Tofu muesli cereal*
Orange
Herbal fruit tea

Whole grain bread
Almond butter (raw)
Raisins
Prune juice

Cream of rye with raisins
Soy or nut milk*
Banana
Molasses tea

Corn bread
Trail mix*
Orange juice

Lunch and Dinner

These menus give you a variety of ways to organize your meals. Use them as guidelines to design your own meal plans. All these dishes were chosen because they contain many nutrients helpful for anemia and heavy menstrual bleeding. See my upcoming cookbook, *Food for Healthy Women*, for more menus and many healthful recipes for women. Starred (*) recipes are included in the following section.

Soup Meals	Vegetable Meals
Navy bean soup	Steamed mixed vegetables:
Corn bread	cauliflower, broccoli, onions,
Mixed green salad	carrots, and green peas
Applesauce	with millet
	Dressing: flax or olive oil
Lentil soup*	Nonsalt seasoning
Mixed grain bread	
Beet, radish, and	Iron-rich taco*
cucumber salad	Dressing: low-salt salsa
Dried figs	
	Guacamole (avocado dip)
Vegetable and lentil soup*	Corn tortillas
Steamed kale	Fresh vegetables to dip
Green beans	
Dried apricots with almonds	Tofu and millet stir-fry*
	Dressing: low-salt soy sauce
Squash and potato soup*	
Steamed spinach	
Broccoli with lemon juice	
Dried pears	

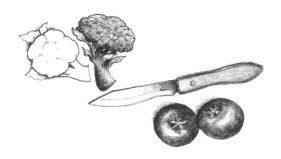

Salad Meals

Iron-rich vegetable salad*
Dressing: oil and vinegar
Whole wheat crackers

Iron-rich fruit salad*
Celery sticks
Rye muffins

Carrot and raisin salad*
Whole grain crackers
Almond butter (raw)

Cole slaw*
Dressing: oil and vinegar
Baked potato with flax oil

Meat Meals

Sautéed liver and onions*
Steamed green beans
Rice
Mixed green salad

Grilled shrimp
Wild rice
Brussels sprouts

Poached salmon*
Brown rice
Steamed asparagus

Poached scallops
Mixed green salad

Note: Try to prepare your cooked dishes with an iron frying pan or skillet. Iron from the skillet will be absorbed by the food. This adds additional supplemental iron for those women with iron deficiency.

Recipes

Beverages

Molasses Tea   *Serves 1*

2 teaspoons blackstrap
   molasses
1 cup warm water

Combine molasses and warm water. Stir thoroughly and serve.

Ginger Tea   *Serves 4*

2 tablespoons grated
   ginger
1 quart water

Add ginger to the water in a cooking pot. Bring to a boil and then turn down the heat to low. Steep for 15 or 20 minutes. Serve with your favorite sweetener.

Fruit Shake   *Serves 1*

1 cup apple juice
2 bananas
1 cup blackberries, blue-
   berries, or strawberries
1/2 cup nondairy milk

Combine apple juice, bananas, berries, and nondairy milk in a blender. Blend until smooth and serve.

Flax Shake   *Serves 1*

6 tablespoons raw flax seeds
1 banana
2 dates, seedless
6 oz. water
4 oz. apple juice

Grind flax seeds to a powder using a coffee or seed grinder. Place powdered flax seeds in a blender. Add remaining ingredients and blend.

Almond Milk   *Makes 1-1/4 cups*

1/2 cup raw or blanched
   almonds
1 tablespoon honey or rice
   syrup
1 cup warm water

Combine nuts, honey, and 1/2 cup of warm water in a blender. Slowly add remaining water and blend until creamy. If you like thinner milk, add 1 to 3 ounces more warm water.

Cereals

Flax Cereal   *Serves 1*

6 tablespoons raw flax
    seed powder
4 oz. apple juice
1/4 teaspoon cinnamon
1 oz. raisins

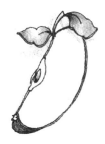

Place raw flax seeds in a seed or coffee grinder. Grind into a powder. Place powder in a cereal bowl and slowly add apple juice and cinnamon, stirring the mixture together. The flax mixture will thicken to a texture like cream of rice or oatmeal. Sprinkle raisins on the cereal. Eat the mixture right away because flax seeds are sensitive to light, air, and temperature. Do not cook this cereal; eat it cold. (Flax seeds may be purchased at a health food store and should be refrigerated.)

Tofu Muesli Cereal #1   *Serves 2*

4 oz. soft tofu
1 tablespoon raw flax oil
1 banana
15 raw almonds
2 oz. nondairy milk
1 oz. raisins

Combine all ingredients except raisins in a food processor. Blend until smooth. Pour into a bowl and sprinkle with raisins. (Flax oil may be purchased at your local health food store and has a delicious nutty flavor. If flax oil is not available in your area, the recipe can be made without it.)

Tofu Muesli Cereal #2   *Serves 2*

4 oz. soft tofu
2 tablespoons ground
    flax seed
1 banana
15 raw almonds
6 strawberries
2 oz. nondairy milk

Combine all ingredients in a food processor. Blend until smooth. Pour into a bowl. (The use of strawberries increases the amount of vitamin C and helps the absorption of iron from the tofu, flax seeds, and almonds.)

All-Bran Cereal   *Serves 1*

1 oz. All-Bran cereal
4 oz. nondairy milk
   (soy, potato, almond)
1 oz. raisins

Combine cereal, nondairy milk, and raisins. (Strawberries may be added to increase vitamin C levels and thereby improve the iron absorption of this high-iron cereal.)

Millet Cereal   *Serves 2*

1 cup millet
2 cups water
1 teaspoon canola oil
4 oz. vanilla soy milk
1 tablespoon honey
1 oz. sunflower seeds
1/2 apple, diced

Wash millet with cold water. Combine millet, water, and canola oil in a cooking pot. Bring ingredients to a rapid boil. Turn flame to low; cover and cook without stirring about 25 to 35 minutes, until millet is soft. Resist the temptation to check before 20 minutes, since that lets out too much steam. Fluff up the millet and spoon into serving bowls. Add the remaining ingredients, mix, and serve.

Spreads

Tofu and Sesame Butter Spread

1/2 cup tofu, drained
1 cup raw sesame butter
1 to 2 tablespoons honey

Makes 1-1/2 cups

Blend all ingredients in a blender or food processor.

Sesame-Almond Butter

1/4 cup soft tofu,
   drained
1/4 cup raw sesame
   butter
6 tablespoons raw
   almond butter
1/8 cup honey

Makes 1-1/2 cups

Combine all ingredients in a blender.

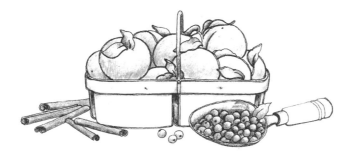

Snacks

Trail Mix #1 *Makes 1-1/2 cups*

1/2 cup raw unsalted
   pumpkin seeds
1/2 cup raw unsalted
   sunflower seeds
1/2 cup raisins

Combine and store in a container in the refrigerator. (This trail mix recipe is very high in iron and other essential nutrients. I use it for a snack food to replace stressful and unhealthy sugar-based sweets and chocolate. It is a great mix to take on trips and I eat it often for breakfast.)

Trail Mix #2 *Makes 1 cup*

1/2 cup dried apricots
1/2 cup raw unsalted
   sunflower seeds
2 tablespoons raw
   sesame seeds

Combine and store in a container in the refrigerator. (This trail mix recipe is also very high in iron and other essential nutrients. Like the preceding recipe, I use it for a snack food to replace stressful and unhealthy sugar-based sweets and chocolate.)

Soups

Squash and Potato Soup

Serves 6

4 summer squash (crook-
neck), sliced
1 potato, diced
1 onion, chopped
3 cups water
1/2 teaspoon low-salt
soy sauce or salt
substitute
1 teaspoon thyme
1/8 bunch parsley,
minced

Steam squash, potatoes, and onions; then, combine the vegetables in a pot. Add the water and cook on low heat with the pot covered for 15 minutes. Add low-salt soy sauce and thyme and continue cooking for another 15 minutes, until vegetables are soft. Let cook and then puree in blender. Garnish with the minced parsley.

Vegetable and Lentil Soup

Serves 4 to 6

3 tomatoes, diced
1/2 cup lentils
1 onion, chopped
1 turnip, chopped
1/2 leek, chopped
1/2 cup green peas
2 carrots, chopped
8 mushrooms, sliced
1/2 tablespoon fennel
1 bay leaf
1/2 tablespoon thyme
1/2 tablespoon oregano
1-1/2 quarts water
1/2 teaspoon salt substitute
1/4 bunch parsley, chopped

Place all ingredients in a pot. Cover with the water. Bring to a boil, then turn heat to low. Cook for 2 hours. Pour the soup into individual serving dishes. Garnish with chopped parsley.

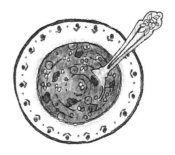

Lentil Soup *Serves 4*

1 cup lentils
1/2 onion, chopped
1/2 cup chopped carrots
1 to 1-1/2 quarts water
1/2 teaspoon low-salt soy
   sauce or salt substitute
1/2 teaspoon thyme

Wash lentils. Put all ingredients in a pot. Bring to a boil, then turn heat to low, cover pot, and simmer for 45 minutes or until lentils are soft.

Split Pea Soup *Serves 4*

1 cup split peas
1/2 onion, chopped
1 small carrot, sliced
1 quart water
1/4 to 1/2 teaspoons sea salt
   or salt substitute
1/2 teaspoon oregano

Wash peas. Place all ingredients in a pot. Bring to a boil, then turn heat to low and cover pot. Cook for 45 minutes or until peas are soft.

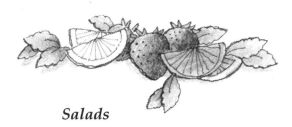

Salads

Iron-Rich Fruit Salad *Serves 4*

1/2 cantaloupe, cubed
16 strawberries
2 bananas, sliced
1 cup cubed pineapple
1/2 cup raisins
4 lettuce leaves

Combine fruit in a large serving bowl. Mix gently. Spoon mixture onto lettuce leaves and serve.

Iron-Rich Vegetable Salad

1 head green or red leaf
    lettuce, torn into pieces
1 large tomato, cut into
    wedges
6 mushrooms, sliced
2 green onions, chopped
6 ounces cooked kidney
    beans
1 avocado, sliced
1/4 cup raw sunflower seeds

Serves 4-6

Combine all ingredients in a large salad bowl. Serve with your favorite dressing.

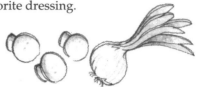

Cole Slaw   *Serves 4*

1/2 teaspoon celery seeds
1/2 teaspoon poppy seeds
1/2 teaspoon dill seeds
2 cups finely shredded red
    cabbage
1-1/2 cups finely shredded
    green cabbage

Crush or grind the seeds and add to shredded cabbage. Serve with favorite dressing (oil and vinegar or honey dressing preferred). (The herbs used are high in iron.)

Potato Salad   *Serves 6*

8 medium-sized red
    potatoes
1 cup chopped celery
1/2 cup finely chopped
    parsley
1/2 cup chopped green
    pepper
1/2 cup chopped sweet,
    raw onions

Steam potatoes for approximately 45 minutes. Cool and cube. Combine celery, parsley, pepper, and onions with potatoes, and mix thoroughly. Add a small amount of your favorite dressing. (Both vinaigrette and low-calorie mayonnaise are delicious on potato salad.)

Carrot-Raisin Salad   *Serves 2*

3 carrots
1/2 cup raisins
1 tablespoon mayonnaise
1 tablespoon cider vinegar

Peel and grate carrots. Mix carrots and raisins with mayonnaise and cider vinegar.

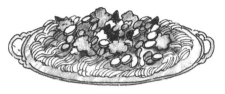

Main Courses

Sautéed Liver and Onions

Serves 4

1 pound calf's liver or
   baby beef liver, organic,
   range-fed
1/2 yellow onion, sliced
2 tablespoons nonwheat
   flour (rice is preferred)
2 tablespoons canola oil

Wipe liver dry and slice. Dip slices in the flour. Heat oil and sauté onions until they begin to brown. Add liver slices, and sauté a few minutes on each side until brown. Reduce heat and cook until liver has reached the preferred level of doneness. Be careful not to overcook as liver will become tough and dry.

Shrimp and Millet Stir-Fry

Serves 4

3/4 cup finely chopped
   celery
1/2 cup water
1 teaspoon sesame or
   safflower oil
1/2 pound shrimp, cooked
   and peeled
3 cups cooked millet
low-salt soy sauce

Sauté celery in water and oil over low heat for 20 minutes or until tender. Add shrimp and cook for 2 minutes. Transfer to a serving dish and toss with millet and low-salt soy sauce to taste.

Tofu and Millet Stir-Fry

Serves 4

3/4 cup cubed tofu
1/4 yellow onion, sliced
1 cup green beans, steamed
1/4 cup water
1 teaspoon sesame or
    safflower oil
3 cups cooked millet
low-salt soy sauce

Combine tofu, onions, and green beans in a large frying pan with water and oil. Cook over low heat for 5 minutes. (Add extra water to pan if needed.) Add millet and mix. Heat for 5 minutes or until warm. Transfer to serving dish and toss with low-salt soy sauce to taste.

Iron-Rich Tacos

Serves 4

4 corn tortillas
3/4 pound pinto beans,
    cooked and pureed
1/2 avocado, thinly sliced
1/4 sweet red pepper, diced
1 tomato, diced
1/4 red onion, finely
    chopped
1/2 head red or romaine
    lettuce, chopped
6 tablespoons salsa

Warm tortillas and beans in separate pans. Place tortillas on individual serving dishes and spread with beans. Garnish with avocado, pepper, tomato, and onion; then cover each taco with lettuce and 1-1/2 tablespoons of salsa.

Poached Salmon

Serves 4

4 fillets of salmon,
    3 oz. each
1 cup water
juice of 1 lemon
1 tablespoon diced onion
1 tablespoon diced carrot

Combine the water and lemon juice in skillet and heat. Place the salmon in the hot liquid and sprinkle with diced vegetables. Cover and poach for 6 to 8 minutes or until the salmon flakes easily with a fork. Remove the fish and keep it warm until you are ready to serve.

Broiled Trout with Dill

Serves 4

2 fresh trout, about
    8 oz. each
2 tablespoons lemon
    juice
chopped fresh dill
    (dried if fresh is
    unavailable)

Slice each trout in half and bone. This will make four fillets. Sprinkle the fillets with lemon juice and dill. Place the trout in a broiler pan. Broil for 5 or 6 minutes or until done.

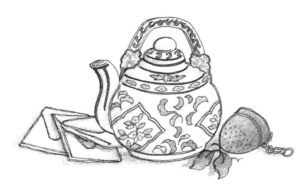

Desserts

Oatmeal Cookies

Makes about 2 dozen

1/2 cup canola oil
1/4 cup honey
1 egg, slightly beaten
2 teaspoons vanilla
1/2 teaspoon salt
1 cup rice flour
3/4 teaspoon baking
    powder
2 cups rolled oats
1 cup raisins

Preheat oven to 375°F. Mix canola oil and honey. Combine with egg, vanilla, and salt and blend. Mix flour, baking powder, rolled oats, and raisins with a fork. Combine all ingredients and mix. A few teaspoons of water may be added until dough is of proper consistency. Spoon onto greased cookie sheets and flatten each cookie slightly with a spoon. Bake for 12 to 15 minutes.

Molasses Cookies

1/2 cup canola oil
1/2 cup honey
1 egg
1/2 cup blackstrap
molasses
1/2 cup soy milk or
nut milk
2-1/2 cups rice flour
1 teaspoon baking soda
1 teaspoon cinnamon
1 teaspoon ginger
1/4 teaspoon salt
1 cup raisins

Makes about 2 dozen

Preheat oven to 350°F. Mix canola oil and honey. Combine with egg, molasses, and soy milk. Mix flour, baking soda, cinnamon, ginger, and salt. Combine all mixed ingredients and blend until batter is smooth. Add raisins and mix well. Drop batter onto a greased cookie sheet. Bake 12 minutes.

Soy milk can be purchased at a health food store. If this is not possible, nut milk can be made easily. See Almond Milk recipe.

Molasses Raisin Bars

6 tablespoons canola oil
1/3 cup honey
2/3 cup blackstrap
molasses
1 egg
1 teaspoon vanilla
1 cup rice flour
1/8 teaspoon salt
1/8 teaspoon baking
soda
1 teaspoon cinnamon
1/8 teaspoon allspice
1/8 teaspoon ginger
1/2 cup raisins

Makes about 20

Preheat oven to 375°F. Mix canola oil and honey. Combine with molasses, egg, and vanilla and blend well. Mix flour, salt, baking soda, cinnamon, allspice, and ginger. Combine all mixed ingredients until batter is smooth. Add raisins to batter and blend well. Pour batter into a well-greased 12 x 18-inch rectangular cake pan (other shapes may be used). Bake for approximately 17 minutes or until center is spongy and cake-like. Cut into bars when cool.

Note: For all dessert recipes, I recommend the use of unsprayed organic raisins. These raisins are available in health food stores. Commercial raisins are among the fruits most heavily sprayed with pesticides.

8

Stress Reduction for Anemia & Heavy Menstrual Flow

*A*nemia and heavy menstrual bleeding seem to cause adverse emotional as well as physical symptoms in many women. Depression can accompany fatigue, and some women note a real decline in zest and energy levels. They complain that as their blood count drops or their menstrual periods become heavier and longer, their joy of living drops, too. Also, because they have less energy, many of these women find that they handle stress less effectively. Small work or family upsets that would normally seem insignificant become magnified. A woman who is tired and has little reserve because of a significant menstrual bleeding problem or anemia may find that major life stresses, such as job loss, death of a loved one, or divorce, seem impossible to deal with.

Exercises for Relaxation

To help you cope with the emotional stresses that may become magnified while you are resolving an anemia or menstrual bleeding problem, I recommend a variety of relaxation methods. Deep breathing, meditation, affirmations, and visualizations can help promote a sense of calm and well-being if practiced on a regular basis. In this chapter I include exercises from all four categories for you to try. Pick those you enjoy most and practice them on a regular basis. I have taught these exercises to women patients and love to practice them myself. Sometimes I recommend that patients learn these techniques on their own through books and tapes; other times I teach the exercises to patients at my office. My patients have been very enthusiastic about the results they attain practicing stress-reduction exercises. They often tell me that they feel much calmer and happier. They also find their physical health has improved. A calm mind seems to have beneficial effects on the body's physiology and chemistry, restoring the body to a normal condition.

First step: Find a comfortable position. For many women, this means lying on their back. You may also do most of the exercises sitting up. Try to keep your spine as straight as possible. Your arms and legs should be uncrossed. It is important that your clothes be loose and comfortable.

Second step: Focus your attention on the exercises; do not allow distracting thoughts to interfere with your concentration. Close your eyes and take a few deep breaths. This will help to quiet your mind and remove your thoughts from the problems and tasks of the day.

Relaxation Methods

Exercise 1: Vitality Breathing

Lie flat on your back with your knees pulled up. Keep your feet slightly apart. Breathe in and out through your nose, if possible.

Inhale deeply. As you breathe in, allow your stomach to relax so that the air flows into your abdomen. Let your stomach balloon out as you breathe in. Visualize the lowest parts of your lungs filling up with air.

Imagine that the air you are breathing in is filled with energy and vitality. Vitality is filling every cell in your body. It fills you with a sensation of warmth and healing. Now, exhale deeply. As you breathe out, imagine the air being pushed out from the bottom of your lungs to the top.

Repeat this sequence until your body feels relaxed and your breathing is slow and regular.

Exercise 2: Color Breathing

Color breathing has traditionally been used to heal the body, calm the nerves, and strengthen the body's energy field. Indian and Oriental spiritual traditions described the body's energy field in detail as far back as 3000 B.C. Intuitives in our culture are able to describe the energy field as lights or colors that emanate from the body.

Different parts of the body appear to emanate different colors: the legs emanate red; the pelvis and intestines, orange; the solar plexus, yellow; the heart, green; the throat, blue; the eyes and pituitary, violet; and the top of the head, white. According to the traditional models, each color gives energy and strength to the body part to which it corresponds.

When you are calm and relaxed, the human energy field looks radiant, harmonious, and full of color. It has the soft, rounded shape of an egg.

Color breathing is a powerful technique to balance the energy field of the body and help heal the systems that are deficient, through a combination of breath work and visualization.

- Sit or lie in a comfortable position. Take a deep breath and imagine that the earth beneath you is filled with the color green. This color goes 50 feet below you into the earth. Imagine that you are opening up energy centers on the bottom of your feet. As you inhale, visualize the beautiful color green (like the green of a park or golf course) filling up your feet. See the bones of your feet filling with green, especially the marrow (or center of the bones) where the red cells are made. See the marrow filling with a beautiful green color. As you inhale, bring the color green up through the center of your leg bones, hip bones, pelvis, spine, ribs, arms, neck, and head. See it flow out of your bones and fill the air around you. Exhale the green slowly out of your lungs. Repeat this process slowly 5 times.

- Now visualize the veins and arteries of your body. They form a network of vessels linking all parts of your body by circulating the blood and oxygen. As you inhale, bring the color red into your blood vessels. Visualize the blood vessels in all parts of your body. The blood vessels of your legs, hips, pelvis, abdomen, chest, arms, neck, and head are filled with bright red. Exhale the red slowly out of your body. See the color fill the air around you. Repeat this process slowly 5 times.

Exercise 3: Meditation

This meditation requires you to sit quietly and engage in a simple and repetitive activity. (This can be very difficult at first.) By emptying your mind, you give yourself a rest. The metabolism of your body slows down. The brain wave slows from the fast beta wave that predominates during the normal working day to a slower alpha or theta wave. This slower pattern is what appears during sleep or in the period of deep relaxation just before falling asleep. Meditating gives the mind a vacation from tension and worry.

- Lie or sit in a very comfortable position.

- Close your eyes and breathe deeply. Let your breathing be slow and relaxed.

- Focus all your attention on your breathing. Notice the movement of your chest and abdomen in and out.

- Block out all other thoughts, feelings, and sensations. If you feel your attention wandering, bring it back to your breathing.

- Count to 1 as you inhale, 2 as you exhale, 3 as you inhale, 4 as you exhale, until you reach 20. Repeat this exercise at least 5 times. For the best results, repeat the sequence for as long as you are able, up to 5 minutes.

Exercise 4: Affirmations for Anemia

The use of affirmations can be a very powerful therapeutic tool when you are embarking on a program to relieve anemia. This is because your state of health is determined by the interaction between your mind and body. You are constantly sending yourself messages—thousands each day—that have a profound effect on your body chemistry and physiology.

I emphasize to all my patients that the body and mind must work together in a positive way for optimal healing to take place. For example, if a patient who has come to me for a weight-loss program has a poor self-image, she will constantly be criticizing herself for the way she looks. This will be reflected in her countenance, posture, mood, and even her ability to follow a beneficial and healthful weight-loss regimen.

The following exercise will help you reprogram yourself toward being anemia-free. Sit in a comfortable position. Repeat the following affirmations three times. Be sure to do this exercise when you are feeling calm and receptive.

- My body is strong and healthy.

- I am anemia-free.

- I produce a normal and healthy amount of red blood cells.

- My bone marrow is healthy; it produces all the red blood cells that I need.

- My red blood cells circulate freely throughout my body.

- My red blood cells contain all the iron I need to carry healthful amounts of oxygen to energize my body.

- My red blood cells carry away all the carbon dioxide waste products easily and efficiently.

- My body is fully oxygenated; my red blood cells pick up abundant oxygen from my lungs.

- I feel fully energized, alive, vital, and strong.

- I have all the stamina and energy I need.

- I eat the food that contains all the nutrients I need for healthy red blood cells.

- My body desires food that is high in essential vitamins and minerals.

- I take time each day to relax and enjoy myself.

- I do a regular, gentle exercise program. I do the exercises that make me feel fully energized and vital.

- I create perfect health within my body.

Exercise 5: Affirmations for Heavy Menstrual Bleeding

- My body is able to regulate its menstrual bleeding pattern.

- I have the perfect amount of menstrual bleeding each month.

- I lose the right amount of blood each month to keep my body healthy.

- I never spot between menstrual cycles.

- I am blood-clot free.

- I have a moderate, comfortable menstrual flow.

- My menstrual cycle comes at the right time each month; I have a regular cycle.

- My ovaries and uterus are healthy.

- My thyroid is healthy and helps regulate my menstrual flow.

- I enjoy my menstrual cycle.

- I eat the food that helps regulate my menstrual flow.

- My body desires food that is high in essential nutrients, vitamins, and minerals.

- I take time each day to relax and enjoy myself.

- I practice the stress-reduction techniques that keep me calm and peaceful.

- I exercise on a regular basis. I do the exercises that I need for a healthy female reproductive tract.

- I create perfect health and well-being within my body.

Exercise 6: Visualization for Anemia

Visualization exercises provide a technique for imagining your body the way you want it to be. This is a very powerful therapeutic tool that I have been using for many years with patients. The technique was pioneered by Carl Simonton, M.D., a cancer radiation therapist, who used this technique with his patients and described the results in his book *Getting Well Again*. He had his patients see their cancers as being small and weak and their immune systems as being big, strong, and capable of destroying the puny cancers (instead of the other way around). He saw many patients go into remission as they visualized their immune systems becoming healthy, using a variety of powerful images such as knights on white horses and jet planes. Visualization exercises can actually let you use imagery to lay down a mental blueprint for a healthier body.

The following visualization exercise for anemia should take several minutes. Feel free to linger on any particular image that pleases you. A successful visualization can actually help trigger the desired healing process in the body.

- Close your eyes. Begin to breathe deeply. Inhale and let the air out slowly. Feel your body begin to relax.

- Imagine that you can look inside your own bones. See the bones of your skull, ribs, chest, and legs. Inside the bones you are making red blood cells. See the red blood cells. They are bright red and shaped like two-sided disks. There are lots of them being formed within your bones. They look strong and healthy.

- As the red blood cells mature, they pass into your blood circulation. See them flowing through your blood vessels so they can reach all parts of your body.

- As they reach your lungs, the red blood cells pick up the oxygen that you have inhaled through your normal, relaxed breathing. See the red blood cells pick up an abundance of life-giving oxygen.

- The red blood cells leave your lungs so they can bring the oxygen to all the tissues of your body. Visualize the oxygen being released and flowing into all your tissues.

- When the oxygen is released, the red blood cells then pick up carbon dioxide, one of your body's primary waste products. Your red blood cells bring your waste products back to the lungs. See your lungs release the carbon dioxide with each breath as you exhale.

- See your body as a vibrating field of energy, full of oxygen and red blood cells. See yourself full of stamina and energy. Your body is in a state of perfect health. Your skin is healthy and clear, your hands and feet are warm, your muscles are relaxed and supple. You feel very calm.

- Now stop visualizing the scene and go back to deep breathing.

- Open your eyes and feel very good.

Exercise 7: Visualization for Heavy Menstrual Bleeding

- Close your eyes. Begin to breathe deeply. Inhale and let the air out slowly. Feel your body begin to relax. Imagine that you can look inside your uterus.

- See the lining of your uterus. It is a lush, blood-rich cushion of tissue.

- Imagine that your uterus is currently in the state that occurs right before your menstrual cycle begins. The blood vessels in the lining of the uterus begin to constrict. See them become coiled and narrow. Visualize them as they begin to release the perfect amount of blood from the uterine lining.

- The blood flows out of the uterus in a moderate, regular flow. See the blood leave the uterus in a steady, healthy manner.

- See the uterine lining slough off into the blood flow so that the uterus can prepare for the next month's cycle.

- Visualize your ovaries and tubes as they connect into the sides of the uterus. Your ovaries are shaped like almonds. They are pink and healthy looking. See them put out healthy levels of your female hormones, estrogen and progesterone. Your ovaries are perfectly regulated and function well each month.

- See the hormones leaving the ovaries to regulate your menstrual flow.

- Now stop visualizing the scene and go back to deep breathing.

- Open your eyes and feel very good.

Putting Your Stress Management Program Together

This chapter has introduced many different ways to help you handle stress better, as well as exercises for improved mind-body health. This can be very useful while you are in the healing stages of anemia and heavy menstrual bleeding. Try each exercise at least once. Experiment with them until you find the combination that works for you. Doing all seven will take no longer than 20 to 30 minutes, depending on how much time you wish to spend with each one. Ideally, the exercises should be done on a daily basis for at least a few minutes each day. Over time, they will help you gain insight into your negative beliefs and change them into positive new ones. Your ability to cope with stress should be tremendously improved.

Suggested Reading

Benson, R., and M. Klipper. *Relaxation Response*. New York: Avon, 1976.

Brennan, B. A. *Hands of Light*. New York: Bantam, 1987.

Davis, M. M., and M. and E. Eshelman. *The Relaxation and Stress Reduction Workbook*. Oakland, CA: New Harbinger Publications, 1982.

Gawain, S. *Creative Visualization*. San Rafael, CA: New World Publishing, 1978.

Gawain, S. *Living in the Light*. Mill Valley, CA: Whatever Publishing, 1986.

Kripalu Center for Holistic Health. *The Self-Health Guide*. Lenox, MA: Kripalu Publications, 1980.

Loehr, J., and J. Migdow. *Take a Deep Breath*. New York: Villard Books, 1986.

Miller, E. *Self-Imagery*. Berkeley, CA: Celestial Arts, 1986.

Ornstein, R., and D. Sobel. *Healthy Pleasures*. Redding, MA: Addison-Wesley, 1989.

9

Exercises for Anemia & Heavy Menstrual Flow

*W*omen who are anemic or have a problem with heavy menstrual bleeding tend to be very tired; they often find that moderate to brisk exercise is difficult for them because they lack stamina and endurance. The fatigue problem tends to resolve as the anemia and bleeding are corrected nutritionally. In the meantime, women with these conditions may completely stop their regular exercise program in an attempt to avoid feeling tired.

However, complete avoidance of exercise is not healthy, for it reduces oxygenation and circulation to vital organs, such as the brain and heart, as well as all the cells of the body. Gentle exercise such as deep breathing exercises, progressive muscle relaxation, range-of-motion exercises to keep the joints mobile, and slow relaxed walking promote good oxygenation and circulation and can even help to increase energy. The key is to exercise in a gentle, slow fashion.

I have included in this chapter several general fitness and flexibility exercises you can use to promote health and well-being. You may want to combine them with gentle aerobic exercise like walking. You can also combine them with the yoga stretches and acupressure points described in Chapters 10 and 11.

Exercise Techniques

Exercise 1: Deep Breathing

Deep, slow abdominal breathing is very important for your health and vitality. It expands your lungs and allows you to bring adequate oxygen, the fuel for metabolic activity, to all the tissues of your body. Rapid, shallow breathing decreases your oxygen supply and keeps you devitalized. Deep breathing helps to relax the entire body and strengthens the muscles in the chest and abdomen. Women with anemia and heavy menstrual bleeding have reduced hemoglobin and red blood cell counts, so less oxygen is available than under normal conditions.

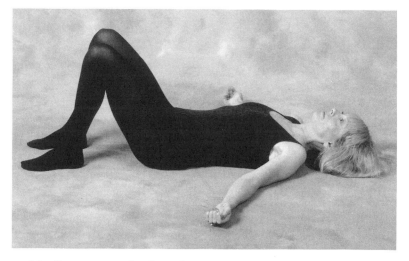

- Lie flat on your back with your knees pulled up. Keep your feet slightly apart. Try to breathe in and out through your nose.

- Inhale deeply. As you breath in, allow your stomach to relax so that the air flows into your abdomen. Your stomach should balloon out as you breathe in. Visualize your lungs filling up with air so that your chest swells out.

- Imagine that the air you breathe is filling your body with energy.

- Exhale deeply. As you breathe out, let your stomach and chest collapse. Imagine the air being pushed out, first from your abdomen and then from your lungs.

Exercise 2: Progressive Muscle Relaxation

Women who are anemic may have muscles that are tense and tight because of inadequate oxygenation and blood flow. Lactic acid tends to accumulate in these muscles, and muscle tension can become a chronic problem. Movement effectively breaks up this pattern of chronically tight muscles. Unfortunately, women with anemia tend to become less active as their fatigue worsens. While strenuous exercise may be too difficult for a woman with anemia, it is still very important to keep the muscles loose and limber. Besides feeling more relaxed, supple muscles have a beneficial effect on mood and induce a sense of peace and calm. The following exercise will aid in releasing muscle tension.

- Lie in a comfortable position. Allow your arms to rest limply, palms down, on the surface next to you. Practice your deep abdominal breathing as you do this exercise.

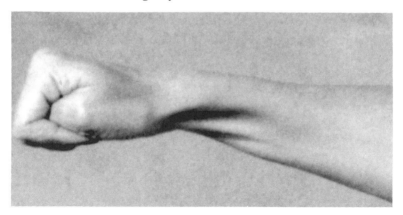

- Clench your hands into fists and hold them tightly for 15 seconds. As you do this, relax the rest of your body. Then let your hands relax.

- Now, tense and relax the following parts of your body in this order: face, shoulders, back, stomach, pelvis, legs, feet, and toes. Hold each part tensed for 15 seconds and then relax your body for 30 seconds before going on to the next part.

- Visualize the tense part contracting, becoming tighter and tighter. On relaxing, see the energy flowing into the entire body like a gentle wave, making all the muscles soft and pliable.

- Finish the exercise by shaking your hands. Imagine the remaining tension flowing out of your fingertips.

Exercise 3: Joint Flexibility

It is very important that women with anemia and heavy menstrual bleeding maintain full range of motion and flexibility in all the joints of the body to reduce the tendency of muscle tension. The following exercise helps to stretch and release tension in the muscles around the joints. This exercise is similar to the "range-of-motion" sequence that physicians may use when testing a patient for joint limitations such as arthritis produces. The exercises are also thought to stimulate the acupuncture meridians as based on the work of Motoyama, a Japanese researcher. In his book, *Theories of the Chakras: Bridge to Higher Consciousness*, Motoyama discusses the importance of these exercises in opening the acupuncture meridians.

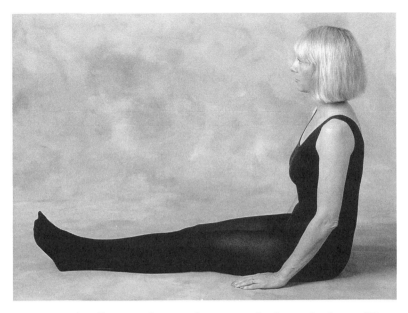

Sit on the floor with your legs stretched out in front. Place your hands at your sides.

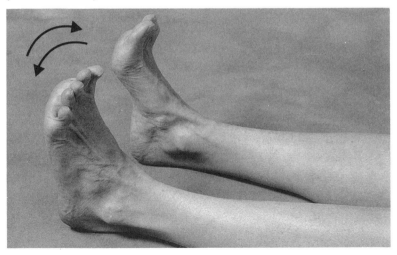

Toes: Slowly flex and extend the toes without moving your feet or ankles. Repeat 10 times.

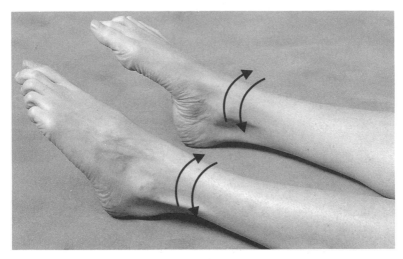

Ankles: Slowly flex and extend the ankle joints. Repeat 10 times. Separate your legs slightly, then rotate your ankles in each direction 10 times. Be sure to keep your heels on the floor.

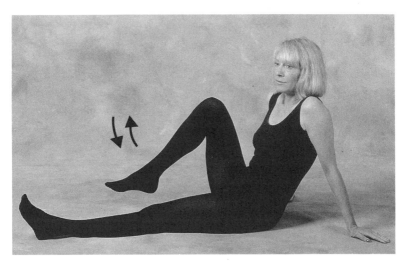

Knees: Still resting in the sitting position, bend the right leg at the knee, bringing the heel near the right buttock. Then lift the right leg off the floor, straightening the right knee. Repeat 10 times. Then do the same exercise with the left leg.

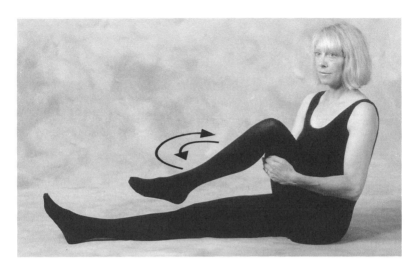

Hold the thigh near the chest with both hands. Rotate your lower leg in a circular motion about the knee 10 times clockwise and then 10 times counterclockwise. Repeat with the left leg.

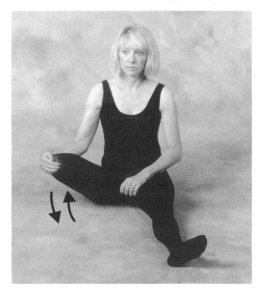

Hips: Bend the right leg so that you can place your right foot on the left thigh. Hold the right knee with the right hand and hold the right ankle with the left hand. Then gently move the right knee up and down with the right hand. Repeat with the left leg.

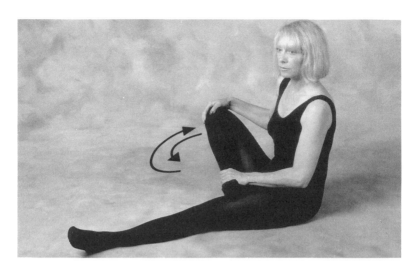

While you are sitting in the same position, rotate the right knee clockwise 10 times and then counterclockwise 10 times. This improves the flexibility of the hip joints. Repeat on the left side.

While sitting, bring the soles of the feet together, bringing the heels close to the body. Using your hands, gently push the knees to the floor and then let them come up again. Repeat 10 times.

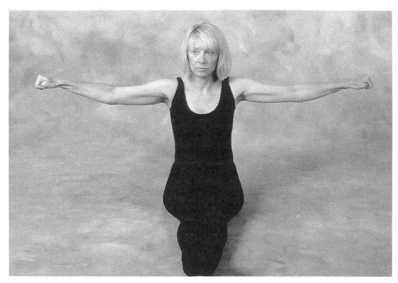

Fingers: Sit on the floor with your legs stretched out in front of you. Lift your arms up to shoulder height, keeping them straight. Open your hands wide. Flex the fingers, closing them over the thumbs to make a fist. Repeat 10 times.

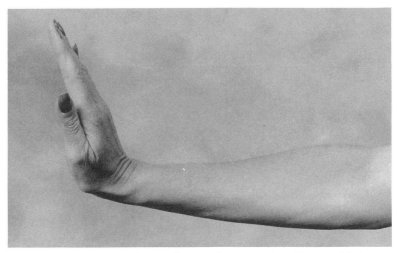

Wrists: Flex and extend your wrists. Repeat 10 times.

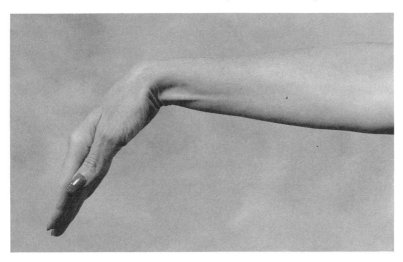

Sitting in the same position, rotate your wrists clockwise and counterclockwise. Repeat 10 times.

Sitting in the same position, hold your hands in extension and move each hand from side to side at the wrist. Repeat 10 times.

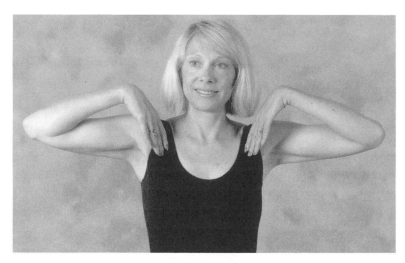

Elbows: Remaining in the same position, stretch out your arms at shoulder height with the palms facing upward. Then bend your arms at the elbow so that your fingers touch the shoulders, and straighten out your arms again. Repeat 10 times with arms extended sideways and ten times with arms facing forward.

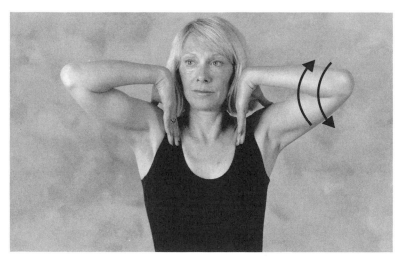

Shoulders: From the same sitting position, with your arms bent and fingertips touching the shoulders, make a circular motion with your elbows. Repeat 10 times clockwise and 10 times counterclockwise.

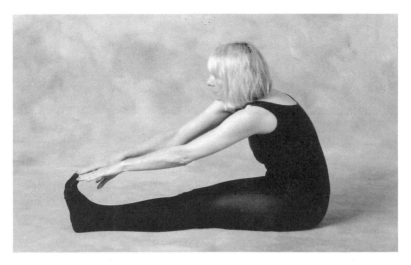

Spine: Remain sitting with your legs together straight out in front of you. Reach over and touch your legs or, without straining, your toes without bending your knees. Repeat 10 times.

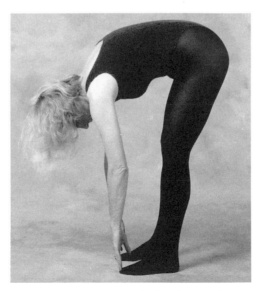

Waist: Stand up and slowly reach over and touch your lower legs or, without straining, your toes as you bend at the waist. Try to keep your knees straight. Repeat 10 times. If you have lower back problems do these two positions with caution.

Suggested Reading

Caillet, R., M.D., and L. Gross. *The Rejuvenation Strategy*. New York: Pocket Books, 1987.

Hanna, T. *Somatics*. Reading, MA: Addison-Wesley, 1988.

Huang, C. A. *Tai Ji*. Berkeley, CA: Celestial Arts, 1989.

Jerome, J. *Staying Supple*. New York: Bantam Books, 1987.

Kripalu Center for Holistic Health. *The Self-Health Guide*. Lenox, MA: Kripalu Publications, 1980.

McLish, R., and V. Joyce, Ph.D. *Perfect Parts*. New York: Warner Books, 1987.

Pinkney, C. *Callanetics: 10 Years Younger in 10 Hours*. New York: Avon, 1984.

Principal, V. *The Body Principal*. New York: Simon & Schuster, 1983.

Tobias, M., and M. Stewart. *Stretch and Relax*. Tucson, AZ: The Body Press, 1985.

Yoga for Anemia & Heavy Menstrual Flow

10

*I*n this chapter I present a series of specific yoga poses that will gently stretch every muscle in your body and will energize and balance the female reproductive tract, breasts, thyroid, and endocrine system. These poses also help optimize the health and well-being of the digestive tract, nervous system, circulation, and all other organ systems of the body. For those women whose anemia is due to dysfunctional menstrual bleeding, which can be worsened by hormonal imbalance and nutritional deficiencies, these poses will provide the benefits of promoting oxygenation and better circulation to the pelvic area. This can have a beneficial effect on menstrual function. The poses will also help reduce muscle tension in the pelvic area. An added benefit for women who are fatigued, due to anemia, can be an increase in vigor and stamina. I do yoga stretches frequently as part of my own exercise routine.

General Techniques for Yoga

When doing yoga exercises, it is important that you focus and concentrate on the positions. First, let your mind visualize how the exercise is to look, and then follow with the correct body placement in the pose. The exercises are done through slow, controlled stretching movements. This slowness allows you to have greater control over your body movements. You minimize the possibility of injury and maximize the benefit to the particular part of the body to which your attention is being directed.

Pay close attention to the initial instructions when beginning an exercise. Look at the placement of the body as shown in the photographs. This is very important, for if the pose is practiced properly, you are much more likely to have relief of your symptoms.

Remember the following as you begin these exercises:

- Try to visualize the pose in your mind, then follow with proper placement of the body.

- Move slowly through the pose. This will help promote flexibility of the muscles and prevent injury.

- Follow the breathing instructions provided in the exercise. Most important, do not hold your breath. Allow your breath to flow in and out easily and effortlessly.

If you practice these yoga stretches regularly in a slow, unhurried fashion, you will gradually loosen your muscles, ligaments, and joints. You may be surprised at how supple you can become over time. If you experience any pain or discomfort, you have probably overreached your current ability and should immediately reduce the amount of the stretching until you can proceed without discomfort. Be careful, as muscular injuries can take quite a while to heal. If you do strain a muscle, I have found that immediately applying ice to the injured area for 10 minutes is quite helpful. Continue to use the ice pack two to three times a day for several days. If the pain persists, see your doctor immediately.

If you want more background and information on yoga, refer to the books listed at the end of this chapter.

Yoga Techniques

Stretch 1: The Pump

This exercise improves blood circulation through the pelvis and thereby stabilizes menstrual function. It helps to calm anxiety and also strengthens the back and abdominal muscles.

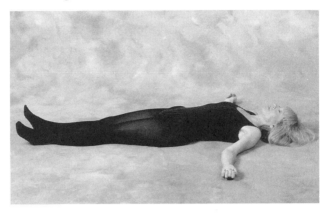

- Lie down and press the small of your back into the floor. This permits you to use your abdominal muscles without straining your lower back.

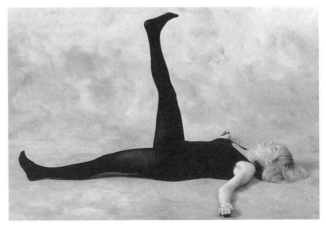

- Raise your right leg slowly while breathing in. Keep your back flat on the floor and let the rest of your body remain relaxed. Move your leg very slowly; imagine your leg being pulled up smoothly by a spring. Do not move your leg in a jerky manner. Hold for a few breaths. Lower your leg and breathe out.

- Repeat the same exercise with your left leg. Then alternate legs, repeating the exercise 5 to 10 times.

Stretch 2: Spinal Flex

This exercise energizes and rejuvenates the female reproductive tract and tones the abdominal organs (pancreas, liver, and adrenals). It emphasizes freer pelvic movement with controlled breathing.

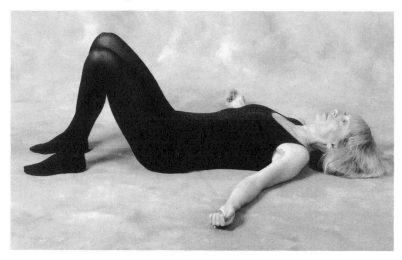

- Lie on your back with your knees bent and your feet on the floor close to your buttocks.

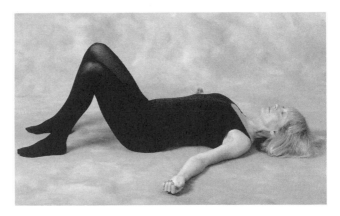

- Exhale and press the lower back into the floor, raising the buttocks slightly.

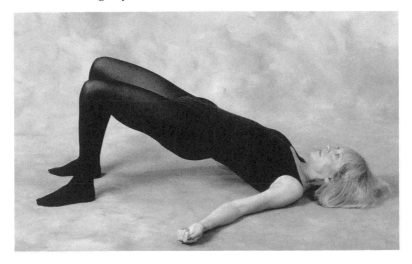

- Arch the back slightly.

- Inhale and lift your lower back off the floor. This stretches the region from the sternum to the pelvis.

- Repeat this exercise 10 times. Always lift your navel up on the in-breath. Always elongate your spine and press the lower back down on the out-breath.

Stretch 3: The Locust

This exercise energizes the entire female reproductive tract, thyroid, liver, intestines, and kidneys. It may be helpful for women with anemia due to dysfunctional bleeding by improving circulation and oxygenation to the pelvic region. This exercise also strengthens the lower back, abdomen, buttocks, and legs, and prevents lower back pain and cramps.

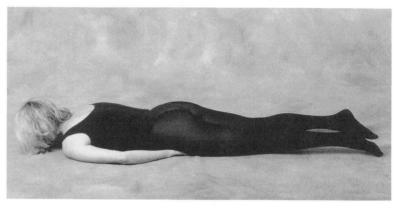

- Lie face down on the floor. Make fists with both your hands and place them under your hips. This prevents compression of the lumbar spine while doing the exercise.

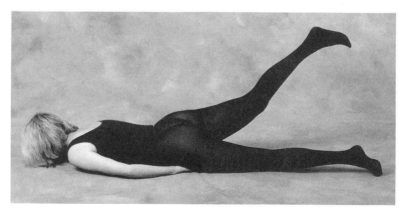

- Straighten your body and raise your right leg with an upward thrust as high as you can, keeping your hips on your fists. Hold for 5 to 20 seconds if possible.

- Lower the leg and slowly return to your original position. Repeat with the left leg, then with both legs together. Remember to keep your hips resting on your fists. Repeat 10 times.

Stretch 4: The Bow

This exercise helps to relieve anemia-related fatigue and lack of vitality, elevating your mood and improving stamina. This exercise also stretches the entire spine and helps to relieve lower back pain and cramps. It stretches the abdominal muscles and strengthens the back, hips, and thighs. It also stimulates the digestive organs and endocrine glands.

- Lie face down on the floor, arms at your sides.

- Slowly bend your legs at the knees and bring your feet up toward your buttocks.

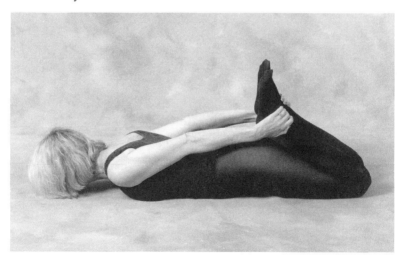

- Reach back with your arms and carefully take hold of first one foot and then the other. Flex your feet to make grasping them easier.

- Inhale and raise your trunk from the floor as far as possible and lift your head. Bring your knees as close together as possible.

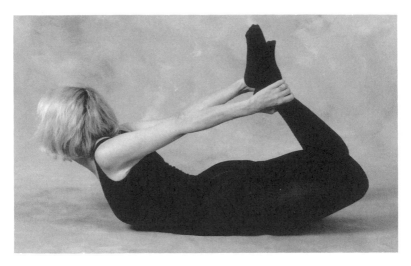

- Squeeze the buttocks while raising them off the floor. Imagine your body looking like a gently curved bow. Hold for 10 to 15 seconds.

- Slowly release the posture. Allow your chin to touch the floor and finally release your feet and return them slowly to the floor. Return to your original position. Repeat 5 times.

Stretch 5: Wide-Angle Pose

This exercise opens the entire pelvic region and energizes the female reproductive tract. It is helpful for varicose veins and improves circulation in the legs.

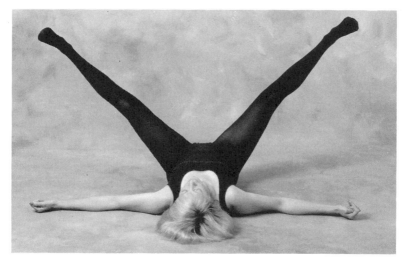

- Lie on your back with your legs against the wall and extended out in a V or an arc, and your arms extended to the side.

Hips should be as close to the wall as possible, buttocks on the floor. Legs should be spread apart as far as they can and still remain comfortable. Breathing easily, hold for 1 minute, allowing the inner thighs to relax.

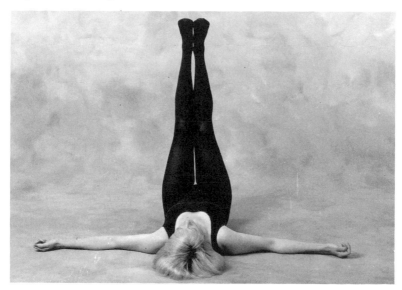

- Bring legs together and hold for 1 minute.

Suggested Reading

Bell, L., and E. Seyfer. *Gentle Yoga*. Berkeley, CA: Celestial Arts, 1987.

Couch, J., and N. Weaver. *Runner's World Yoga Book*. New York: Runner's World Books, 1979.

Folan, L. Lilias, *Yoga, and Your Life*. New York: McMillan Publishing Co., 1981.

Iyengar, B.K.S. *Light on Yoga*. New York: Schocken Books, 1966.

Mittleman, R. *Yoga 28 Day Exercise Plan*. New York: Workman Publishing Co., 1969.

Moore, M., and M. Douglas. *Yoga*. Arcane, ME: Arcane Publications, 1967.

Singh, R. *Kundalini Yoga*. New York: White Lion Press, 1988.

Stearn, J. *Yoga, Youth and Reincarnation*. New York: Bantam, 1965.

11

Acupressure for Anemia & Heavy Menstrual Flow

$\mathcal{A}$cupressure is an easy-to-use method of applying finger pressure to specific points on the body in order to help prevent disease and illness. It has been an important part of traditional Oriental healing for many centuries and is often used along with herbs to promote healing.

Acupressure is based on the belief that there exists within the body a life energy or "biofield." This life energy is called *chi*. It is different from, yet similar to, electromagnetic energy. Health is thought to be a state in which the chi is equally distributed throughout the body and is present in sufficient amounts. It is thought to energize all the cells and tissues of the body.

The life energy is thought to run through the body in channels called *meridians*. When working in a healthy manner, these channels distribute the energy evenly throughout the body, sometimes on the surface of the skin and at times deep inside the body, in the organs. Disease occurs when the energy flow in a meridian is blocked or stopped. As a result, the internal organs that correspond to the meridians can show symptoms of disease. The meridian flow can be corrected by stimulating the points on the skin surface. These points can be treated easily by hand massage. When the normal flow of energy through the body is resumed, the body is believed to heal itself spontaneously.

Stimulation of the acupressure points through finger pressure can be done by you or by a friend following simple instructions. It is safe, painless, and does not require the use of needles. It can be used without the years of specialized training needed for insertion of acupuncture needles.

How to Perform Acupressure

- Acupressure may be done either by yourself or by a friend when you are relaxed. Your room should be warm and quiet. Hands should be clean and nails trimmed to avoid bruising. If your hands are cold, warm them in water.

- Choose the side of the body to work on that has the most discomfort. If both sides are equally uncomfortable, choose whichever one you want. Working on one side seems to relieve the symptoms on both sides. There appears to be a transfer of energy or information from one side to the other.

- Hold each point indicated in the exercise with a steady pressure for 1 to 3 minutes. Pressure should be applied slowly with the tips or balls of the fingers. It is best to place several fingers over the area of the point. If you feel resistance or tension in the area on which you are applying pressure, you may want to push a little harder. However, if your hand starts to feel tense or tired, lighten the pressure a bit. Make sure that your hand is comfortable. The acupressure point may feel somewhat tender. This means that the energy pathway or meridian is blocked.

- During the treatment, the tenderness in the point should slowly go away. You may also have a subjective feeling of energy radiating from this point into the body. Many patients describe this sensation as very pleasant. Don't worry if you don't feel it—not everyone does. The main goal is relief from your symptoms.

- Breathe gently while doing each exercise.

- The point that you are to hold is shown in the photograph accompanying the exercise. All these points correspond to specific points on the acupressure meridians.

- Massage the points once a day or more during the time that you have symptoms.

Acupressure Exercises

Exercise 1:
Balances the Reproductive System

This exercise normalizes the energy of the reproductive organs by balancing points on the bladder meridian. It also relieves lower back pain and can help to relieve excessive menstrual bleeding.

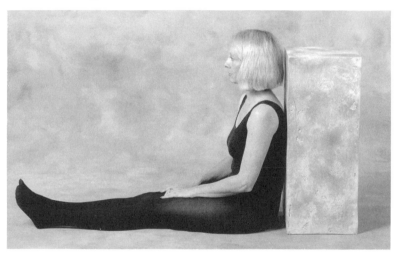

- Sit on the floor and prop your back against a wall or a heavy piece of furniture. Hold each step for 1 to 3 minutes.

Alternative method: Lie on the floor and put your lower legs over the seat of a chair. Follow the exercise from that position.

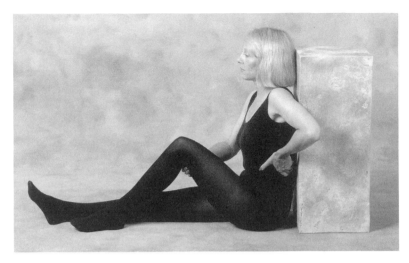

- Place left hand 1 inch above the waist on the muscle to the left side of the spine (muscle will feel firm and rope-like).

  Place right hand behind crease of the left knee.

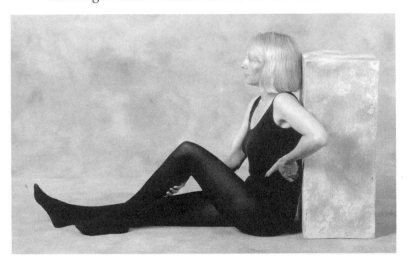

- Left hand stays in the same position.

  Right hand is placed on the center of the back of the left calf. This is just below the fullest part of the calf.

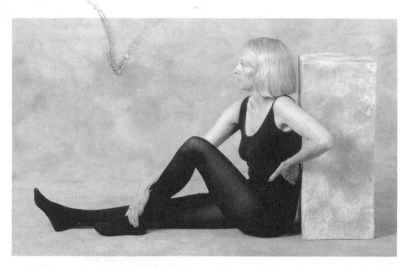

- Left hand remains 1 inch above the waist on the muscle to the side of the spine.

  Right hand is placed just below the ankle bone on the outside of the left heel.

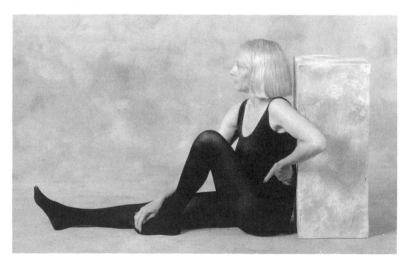

- Left hand remains 1 inch above the waist on the muscle to the side of the spine.

  Right hand holds the front and back of the left little toenail.

Exercise 2:
Relieves Excessive Menstrual Bleeding

This exercise has been used traditionally in controlling excessive uterine bleeding.

- Sit upright on a chair. Hold each step for 1 to 3 minutes.

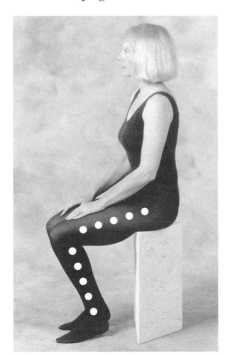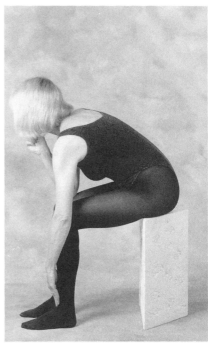

- Bend over at the waist with left hand holding point in front of ankle bone. Move hand slowly along points on leg.

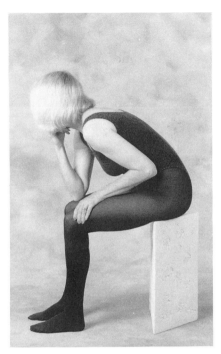 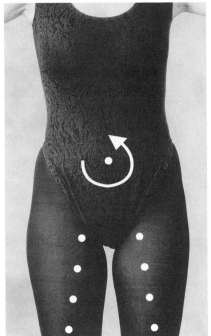

- Move left hand slowly on points to the top of the thigh.
  Repeat on the right side with right hand.

- Right hand in middle of thigh points up to groin. Repeat on
  other side with left hand. Circle area around navel in counterclockwise direction.

Exercise 3:
Relieves Thyroid Imbalance

This exercise energizes the thyroid, which can cause excessive menstrual bleeding and anemia.

- Sit upright on a chair. Hold each step for 1 to 3 minutes.

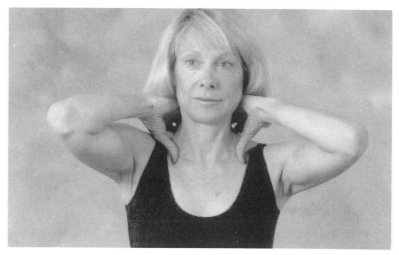

- Wrap hands around shoulders with thumbs pressing gently into both sides on top of collarbone.

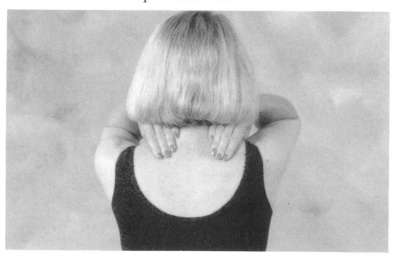

- Fingers are in back and press against upper shoulders and shoulder blade area.

Exercise 4:
Use for Relief of Anemia

This sequence of points is important for the treatment of anemia. It involves the stimulation of points on the spleen meridian that affect blood formation and menstrual problems.

- Sit upright on a chair. Hold each step for 1 to 3 minutes.

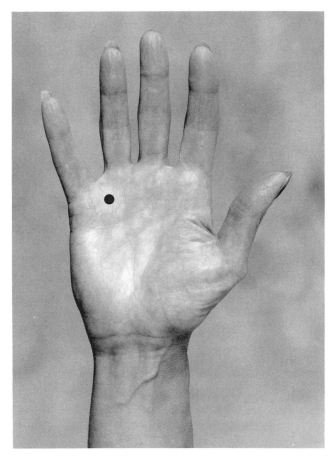

- Left hand holds a point on the right palm below fourth and fifth fingers.

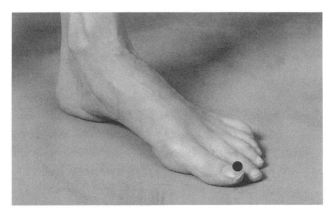

- Left hand holds a point at the inner aspect of the big toe.

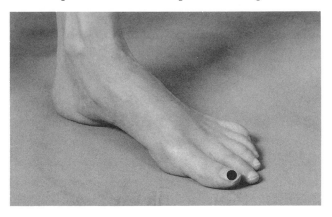

- Left hand holds a point over the nail of the big toe.

Exercise 5:
Use for Relief of Fatigue and Tiredness

This exercise helps to relieve the fatigue and tiredness that commonly accompany anemia and heavy menstrual bleeding.

- Sit upright on a chair. Hold each step for 1 to 3 minutes.

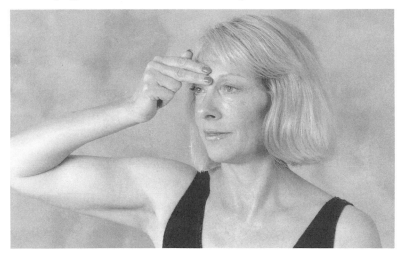

- Right hand holds a point directly between the eyebrows, where the bridge of the nose meets the forehead.

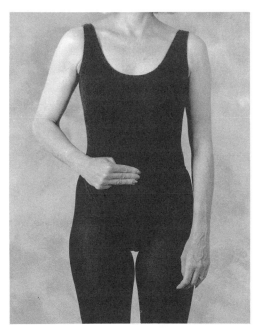

- Fingers hold a point below the navel. Measure three finger-widths below the navel to find this point.

Suggested Reading

The Academy of Traditional Chinese Medicine. *An Outline of Chinese Acupuncture.* New York: Pergamon Press, 1975.

Bauer, C. *Acupressure for Women.* Freedom, CA: The Crossing Press, 1987.

Chang, S. T. *The Complete Book of Acupuncture.* Berkeley, CA: Celestial Arts, 1976.

Gach, M. R., and C. Marco. *Acu-Yoga.* Tokyo: Japan Publications, 1981

Houston, F. M. *The Healing Benefits of Acupressure.* New Canaan, CT: Keats Publishing, 1974.

Kenyon, J. *Acupressure Techniques.* Rochester, VT: Healing Arts Press, 1980.

Nickel, D. J. *Acupressure for Athletes.* New York: Henry Holt, 1984.

Pendleton, B., and B. Mehling. *Relax With Self-Therap/Ease.* Englewood Cliffs, NJ: Prentice Hall, 1984.

Teeguarden, I. *Acupressure Way of Health: Jin Shin Do.* Tokyo: Japan Publications, 1978.

12

How to Put
Your Program
Together

*T*he *Anemia & Heavy Menstrual Flow Self-Help Book* provides a complete self-help program to prevent and relieve your symptoms. The Complete Treatment Chart on page 43 summarizes the many treatment options presented in this book. Use this chart for reference as you devise your own program. Try the treatment options that feel most comfortable to you. You may find, for example, in trying the exercises or the stress-reduction techniques, that certain routines feel better to you than others. If that is the case, practice those that bring the greatest sense of relief for your particular symptoms.

Always keep in mind that your ultimate goal is relief of your anemia or heavy menstrual bleeding problem resulting in a major improvement in your overall health and well-being. I generally recommend beginning any self-help program slowly so that you have the time to get comfortable with the lifestyle changes. Everyone has a different capacity for adjusting to major changes in lifestyle. While some of my patients like to eliminate their old, unhealthy habits as quickly as possible, many other women find such rapid changes in their long-term habits to be too stressful. Find the pace that works for you.

Enjoy the program. I always tell my patients to regard their self-help program as an enjoyable adventure. The exercises and stress-reduction techniques should give you a sense of energy and well-being. The menus and food selections in this book provide you with an opportunity to try delicious and healthful new foods.

As you do the program, don't set unrealistic or too strict expectations for yourself. You don't have to be perfect to get great results. Just follow the guidelines of the program as well as you can and as your schedule permits.

It is not a disaster if you forget to take your vitamins occasionally or don't have time to exercise on any particular day. Don't be discouraged if you can't follow the dietary recommendations on vacations, holidays, and birthdays. Periodically, review the guidelines outlined in this book and continue to adapt your lifestyle to the healthful suggestions that I've shared with you. Over time you will notice many beneficial changes.

Be your own feedback system. Your body will tell you if you are on the right track and if what you are doing is making you feel better. It will also tell you if your diet and emotional stresses are increasing your symptoms. Remember that even moderate changes in your habits can make significant differences.

The Anemia & Heavy Menstrual Flow Workbook

At the start of your program, fill out the workbook section of this book. The workbook questionnaires will help you evaluate which areas in your life have contributed most to your symptoms and need the most work. Use the workbook every month or two as you follow the self-help program. The workbook will help you see the areas in which you are making the most progress, both with symptom relief and with the initiation of healthier lifestyle habits. The workbook can give you organized and easy-to-use feedback on your progress with the program.

Diet and Nutritional Supplements

I recommend that you make all nutritional changes gradually. Many women find breakfast the easiest meal to change because it is simple and often eaten at home. To change your other meals and snacks, periodically review the list of foods to avoid and foods to emphasize. Each month pick a few foods that you are willing to eliminate from your diet. Try the foods that help prevent and relieve anemia and heavy menstrual bleeding. The recipes and menus included in this book should be very helpful as you restructure your diet.

Vitamins, minerals, and herbal supplements can help complete your nutritional needs and speed up the healing process. They are a very important part of the program for most women.

Stress Reduction

The stress-reduction exercises play an important role in facilitating the physical healing process. I find that all my patients heal more rapidly from almost any problem when they are calm, happy, and relaxed. The visualization exercises actually help you set a blueprint in your mind for optimal health. This allows the body and mind to work together in harmony.

Begin the program initially by putting aside 15 to 30 minutes each day, depending on the flexibility of your schedule. Try all the stress-reduction exercises listed in this book. Choose the combination that works best for you. Practice stress management on a regular basis.

You do not need to spend enormous amounts of time on these exercises. Many women are too busy to spend an hour a day meditating. Even 10 minutes out of your daily schedule can be helpful. You may find that the quietest times for you are early in the morning before you get out of bed or late at night before going to sleep. Other women simply choose to take a break during the day. You can close the door to your office or go into your bedroom at home for 10 minutes to relax. Use the time to breathe deeply, do the visualizations, or meditate. You will be much calmer and more relaxed afterward.

Exercise

You should exercise on a regular basis, at least three times a week. Women with anemia or heavy menstrual bleeding may find that vigorous exercise is too stressful and tiring. Follow the gentle stretches and acupressure exercises in this book. Aerobic exercise such as walking should be done slowly and comfortably and never to the point of exhaustion. It is important that women who are tired, because of anemia or heavy menstrual bleeding, keep their muscles and joints flexible and supple. This will help combat fatigue by enhancing circulation to all parts of the body. Try the fitness and flexibility exercises in this book.

To do the stretches and acupressure exercises described in this book, set aside a half-hour each day for the first week or two of your self-help program. Try all the exercises. After an initial period of exploration, choose the ones that you enjoy most and that seem to give you the most relief. Practice them on a regular basis so that they can help prevent and reduce your symptoms.

Conclusion

I wish to reaffirm that each of us can do a tremendous amount for ourselves to assure optimal health and well-being. By having access to information, education, and health resources, every woman can play a major role in creating her own state of good health. Practice the beneficial self-help techniques outlined in this book. Follow good nutritional habits, exercise, and practice regular stress-reduction techniques.

By combining good principles of self-care along with your regular medical care, you can enjoy the same wonderful results that my patients and I have had for a life of good health and well-being.

Health & Lifestyle Resources for Women

The LIFECYCLES Center

Health and lifestyle resources are available to provide women with the information, education, and resources that all women need for optimal health and well-being. For many years, I have been a strong advocate of the need for these resources. When women have access to information about important health issues, they can participate in and promote their own well-being. Having worked with many thousands of women of all ages, both as patients and in my classes, I have been impressed by their intense desire for information on how to stay healthy.

Unfortunately, finding information on major health issues has been difficult for most women. First of all, research on women's health issues has traditionally been a low priority in the medical and scientific community. Very few government dollars have been spent researching the major female health problems. In addition, a woman who is faced with the need to handle a significant female-related problem finds an almost total lack of available information. I receive calls and letters from women all over the world who are searching for self-care resources for a variety of health issues. These necessary resources for women who want to practice good preventive health care and stay healthy are available through *The LIFECYCLES Center.*

Resources Currently Available

The Center provides complete self-help programs and resources for a variety of women's health-care and lifestyle issues, including PMS, menstrual cramps, menopause, anemia, heavy menstrual bleeding, chronic fatigue and tiredness, and back discomfort. Additional self-help programs will be added in 1992 and 1993. Self-help books on weight control, breast cysts and tumors, anxiety and moodiness, and chronic fatigue syndrome will be available soon. I have spent the past 20 years gathering these resources. I use the following techniques and products constantly in my own wellness programs and recommend them for use by my patients. The following top quality resources for women are available:

Books by Susan M. Lark, M.D.
PMS Self-Help Book
Menopause Self-Help Book
Anemia & Heavy Menstrual Flow—A Self-Help Program
Menstrual Cramps—A Self-Help Program
Chronic Fatigue and Tiredness—A Self-Help Program

Tapes
PMS Stress Reduction Tape

Foods
Flax Oil. Flax oil is the best source of the essential fatty acids that are so important for women's optimal reproductive health. This oil has a delicious buttery flavor. Flax oil is delicate and should not be used for cooking, but adds great buttery flavor to popcorn, potatoes, rice, steamed vegetables, pasta, hot cereals, and many other dishes. Add this oil to your food just before serving.

Flax Oil and Borage Capsules. This is a great way to take es-sential fatty acids as a supplement. I recommend that women take at least 4 capsules a day for nutritional support for dry skin and vaginal tissues, PMS cramps, and menopausal symptoms. Fatty acids are found throughout the body and provide important support to maintain optimal health and wellness in many body systems for women. Borage oil is excellent for PMS, cramps and endometriosis nutritional support.

Flax Seed Powder. This makes a delicious cereal base. Just stir in apple juice or milk for a great tasting cereal. You can also sprinkle flax seed powder on cereals, casseroles, and desserts for a delicious nutty flavor.

Nondairy Milk. This new potato-based milk, Vegelicious®, is absolutely fantastic. It contains 240 mg of calcium per 8-ounce serving. I strongly recommend its use for women with any type of menstrual problem, including PMS and menstrual cramps as well as menopause. It is an excellent replacement for cow's milk since it does not contain the chemicals that worsen these common female conditions. It is also a great cow's milk substitute for adults and children with allergies and food sensitivities because it is easy to digest. Children love its taste. Use it for any purpose that you would use milk.

Vitamin & Mineral Supplements Formulated Specifically for Women

I have developed the following formulas that provide complete nutritional support for women who want to practice healthy lifestyle and nutritional habits as part of their treatment program for a variety of common female complaints.

PMS Nutritional System
Menopause Nutritional System
Woman's Daily Spectrum Nutritional System
Women's Daily Iron Nutritional System
Women's Water Balance
Unwind for Relaxation
Bioflavonoids

Herbal Tinctures for Women

The following herbs supply beneficial nutritional support for women. Combine these herbs according to the formula in the book. They are available at the Center in large 4-and 8-ounce sizes. This is the most economical and cost-effective way to purchase herbs.

Yellow dock	Ginger root
Huckleberry	White willow bark
Oregon grape root	Red raspberry leaf
Tumeric	Cramp bark
Wild yam	Chamomile
Shepherd's purse	Hops
Golden seal	Chaste tree berry (Vitex)
Sarsaparilla	Ginkgo biloba
Parsley	Buchu
Black cohosh	

Recipe Cards

The recipe cards and meal plans were developed by me and are based on the knowledge I have gained through my work in the field of women's health care and preventive medicine. Each packet provides women with delicious, easy-to-prepare recipes for meals that contain therapeutic levels of the nutrients women need for good health.

Recipe Cards for Healthy Women—Breakfast
Recipe Cards for Healthy Women—Lunch and Dinner
Recipe Cards for Healthy Women—Snacks and Desserts

Women's Personal Products

Vitamin E Vaginal Suppositories. These suppositories help soothe the vaginal tissues. They are particularly helpful to postmenopausal women for whom vaginal dryness and irritation can be a real source of discomfort.

Products for Back Discomfort

The Archable Body Bridge. A wonderful device that stretches the body naturally along its arc. This is a terrific tool to help increase overall flexibility, correct poor body alignment, and improve posture. Use every day for relaxation and relief of muscle tension. This is a very useful device for women who tend to get menstrual cramps, because it stretches and relaxes tense pelvic and abdominal muscles. This device can be particularly helpful for women who sit for long periods of time when they have menstrual cramps.

Please contact the Center directly if you are interested in obtaining any of the self-help programs or resources for women.

The LIFECYCLES Center
101 First Street, Suite 441
Los Altos, CA 94022-2706
(415) 964-7268 (For information)
(800) 862-9876 (For orders only)

Notes

Product List

The *LIFECYCLES Center*
101 First Street, Suite 441
Los Altos, CA 94022-2706
(415) 964-7268 (For information)
(800) 862-9876 (For orders only)

Books by Susan M. Lark, M.D.

PMS Self-Help Book
Menopause Self-Help Book
Anemia & Heavy Menstrual Flow—A Self-Help Program
Menstrual Cramps—A Self-Help Program
Chronic Fatigue and Tiredness—A Self-Help Program

Tapes

PMS Stress Reduction Tape

Foods

Flax Oil
Flax Oil and Borage Oil Capsules
Flax Seed Powder
Vegelicious Non-Dairy Milk

Vitamin & Mineral Supplements Formulated Specifically for Women

PMS Nutritional System
Menopause Nutritional System
Woman's Daily Spectrum Nutritional System
Women's Daily Iron Nutritional System
Women's Water Balance
Unwind for Relaxation
Bioflavonoids

Herbal Tinctures for Women

Yellow dock
Huckleberry
Oregon grape root
Tumeric
Wild yam
Shepherd's purse
Golden seal
Sarsaparilla
Black cohosh
Buchu

Ginger root
White willow bark
Red raspberry leaf
Cramp bark
Chamomile
Hops
Chaste tree berry
Ginkgo biloba
Parsley

Recipe Cards

Recipe Cards for Healthy Women—Breakfast
Recipe Cards for Healthy Women—Lunch and Dinner
Recipe Cards for Healthy Women—Snacks and Desserts

Women's Personal Products

Vitamin E Vaginal Suppositories

Products for Back Discomfort

The Archable Body Bridge
Please contact the Center directly if you are interested in obtaining any of our self-help programs and resources for women.

About the Author

Susan M. Lark, M.D., is a noted authority in women's health care and preventive medicine and is Director of *The LIFECYCLES Center*. She also maintains a private practice in Los Altos, California. Dr. Lark has been on the clinical faculty of Stanford University Medical School, Department of Family and Preventive Medicine. She is an associate member of the Department of Family Medicine, El Camino Hospital in Mountain View, California. Dr. Lark lectures widely on women's health-care issues and is the author of two best-selling guides for women: *The PMS Self-Help Book* (Celestial Arts) and *The Menopause Self-Help Book* (Celestial Arts).

Women seeking appointments for patient care or information about lectures and speaking engagements can reach Dr. Lark through *The LIFECYCLES Center*. She is also available for phone consultation with women living outside the San Francisco Bay Area who would like more personalized information. Contact Dr. Lark at the Center, (415) 964-7268, for available time and fee schedule.

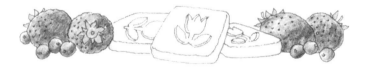

Acknowledgment

The author and publisher wish to extend a special acknowledgment to Shelly Reeves Smith and Cracom Corporation for permission to reproduce the creative line drawings found in the food section of this book. These and additional drawings, together with a collection of wonderful recipes, may be found in the cookbook *Just a Matter of Thyme* available in your local gift or book store. Inquires may be addressed to Among Friends, P.O. Box 1476, Camdenton, MO 65020 or call toll free 1-800-377-3566.

Index